PILLARS OF LIGHT

GODDESS ACTIVATIONS™

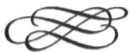

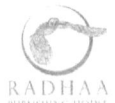

COPYRIGHT

All rights reserved.

No part of this book may be reproduced in any form or by any electronic or mechanical means, including information storage and retrieval systems, without written permission from the author, except for the use of brief quotations in a book review.

Copyright © 2021 by Radhaa Publishing House

Goddess Activations™, Goddess Code™ are Trademark.

Radhaa Publishing House | radhaapublishinghouse.com
    Cover Art by Jon Marro

ISBN: Paperback: 978-1-952124-06-8

CONTENTS

Dedication	v
Foreword	ix
Introduction	xv
Radhaa Nilia	
Chapter 1	1
INTRODUCTION TO GODDESS ACTIVATIONS™	
Chapter 2	11
PERSONAL STORIES of GODDESS ACTIVATIONS™	
About Radhaa Nilia	27
Chapter 3	29
PELE GODDESS ACTIVATIONS™	
Hilda Zamora	35
Chapter 4	37
APHRODITE GODDESS ACTIVATIONS™	
Danielle Schreck	49
Chapter 5	51
LAKSHMI GODDESS ACTIVATIONS™	
Maya Verzonilla	59
Chapter 6	61
SARASWATI GODDESS ACTIVATIONS™	
Anna Lieberman	73
Chapter 7	75
DURGA, MA'AT GODDESS ACTIVATIONS™	
Abigail Diaz Juan	91
Chapter 8	93
SOPHIA GODDESS ACTIVATIONS™	
Alanna Starr Shimel	105
Chapter 9	107
IXCHEL GODDESS ACTIVATIONS™	
Raziel F. Arcega	117
Chapter 10	119
LALITA GODDESS ACTIVATIONS™	
Angelica	129
Chapter 11	131
AKHILANDESHWARI GODDESS ACTIVATIONS™	
Shakti Devi	139
Chapter 12	141
ABUNDANTIA GODDESS ACTIVATIONS™	

Brenda Lainof	149
Chapter 13	151
FREYA GODDESS ACTIVATIONS™	
Y'Shell Esta	165
Chapter 14	167
GREEN TARA GODDESS ACTIVATIONS™	
Michelle Lopez	177
Chapter 15	179
CASSANDRA GODDESS ACTIVATIONS™	
Lori Santo	185
Chapter 16	187
MOTHER MARY GODDESS ACTIVATIONS™	
Kory Muniz	195
Chapter 17	197
BRIGIT GODDESS ACTIVATIONS™	
Michelle L. Casto	203
Chapter 18	205
MARY MAGDALENE GODDESS ACTIVATIONS™	
Blossom Rountree	215
Chapter 19	217
JOURNEY TO THE GODDESS	
Radhaa Nilia	227
ABOUT RADHAA PUBLISHING HOUSE	231

DEDICATION

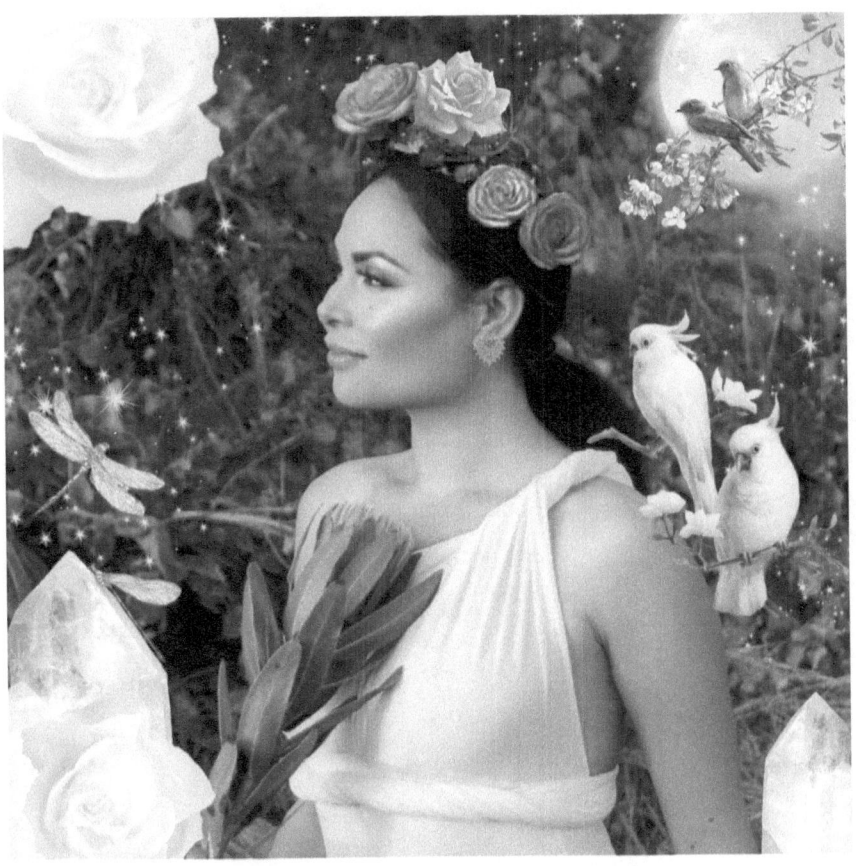

Pillars of Light: Stories of Goddess Activations™ is dedicated to the Goddess in every Woman.

Sister,

You know you have prepared for many lifetimes
to be a part of this Great Awakening on Earth!

The time has come for you to ignite your
Goddess Code and all the gifts that comes with it.
It is part of your divine destiny and Legacy.

Now is the time to break the chains that have
held you down in suffering!

You're here to share your wisdom,
power and be the magical timeline-shifter
that you are.

You are always meant to be a sovereign being,
and the clarion call is here for you
to reclaim the Pillar of your Light.

It is time to raise the
Goddess Pillar of Light within ourselves
and across the World.
Together we RISE.

Wings of Isis,
Awaken the Goddess
Anchor the Codes of Truth
May Justice reign on Earth
We stand as Pillars of Light
The time is Now.

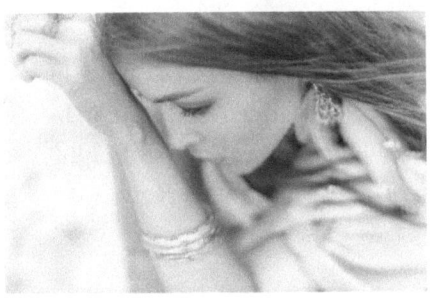

Wings of Isis,
Spread your wings
Wide and far
Awaken the Goddess
In broken hearts of women
Clear the trauma of Genocide
Women burned across the world
Witch hunts that took their lives
Women made guilty
of being authentic
with her heart, her soul, her intuition
A war on Priestess Temples of Light
Who is smashing the Pillars and statures alike?
So afraid of the feminine in her fullness
They removed her from sacred space
Putting dark ones in her place.
Sophia codes inverted,
Everything became distorted.
We are the ones we've been waiting for.

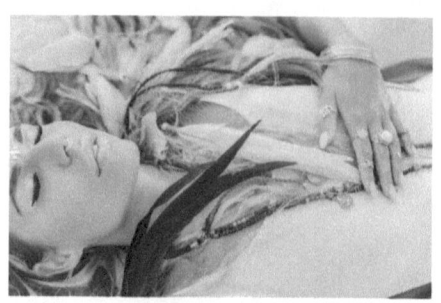

Anchor the Codes of Truth
May Justice reign on Earth
We stand as Pillars of Light
The time is Now.

FOREWORD

MAYA THE SHAMAN

Namaskar Divine One,

 My name is Maya the Shaman, and I am honored to write this foreword for Pillars of Light: Stories of Goddess Activations™. You see, the Goddess has always been a part of my life growing up. I grew up in Laguna, Philippines, near Mount Makiling, the land of the great Goddess named Maria Makiling, Goddess of Nature. There were many Deities, Gods, and Goddesses in our Mythology before the Spanish Inquisition. Like many places in the world, the traditional values of honoring the divine feminine, the Goddesses, were deleted from our culture through Catholic indoctrination. And most of the divine traditions worthy of remembering had indeed been erased in our indigenous cultures alike in our world.

 My family moved to another locality called Cainta, Rizal. Growing up with the peacefulness of a small village, I had witnessed one day a disturbing event when suddenly, our very home and land were taken away by the Church in Valley Golf. The Church had sent out hired gunmen to do the dirty work, knocked on each person's home with the demand to leave our homes at once, not even 24 hours notice, in the name of the Catholic Church. They forcefully displaced women, children, families and instilled great fear in the name of God. They didn't just knock; they knocked with riffles on the doors. When we opened them, they put guns to my father's head and proclaimed that this land had belonged to the Church and we had to get out now! My father resisted, many did, but we had no other weapons to fight with.

Our family and the entire village had to pack that moment as the Churches gunmen watched on with no empathy or remorse as villagers cried on losing their homes. We were forced to take what we could only carry with us and leave all of our belongings behind. With hundreds of people nowhere to go, we were suddenly homeless by Church orders. The entire village was bulldozed. Not a single foundation was left standing of five hundred homes. All of us were grieving in losing what we built and created. The conquerors once again stole what belonged to the people of this land. The severe shock and trauma were overwhelming. It was life and death, a war against injustice. I cannot remember where we slept that night or the nights to come. All I recalled were sobbing mothers, crying children, and screams.

Tears of men who worked their whole lives to provide shelter and food for their families lost hope. Their divine masculine was also stolen and replaced by shame and grief. Not good enough. Worthless. Thieves steal more than just homes. They steal the dignity and honor of honest, hardworking people. And this is what the dark patriarchy has done across the world for centuries, from witch-hunts to indigenous lands. This dark greed to steal all lands, cultures, and divinity, including our disconnection through women's worship to the Goddesses, were crimes against humanity.

It's no wonder HIStory has been so distorted. The conquerors wrote their lies. And so, History must be re-written. And we re-write it by our remembering, our holiness.

"The Gods and Goddesses of myth, legend and fairy tale represent archetypes, real potencies, and potentialities deep within the psyche, which, when allowed to flower, permit us to more fully be human." ~Margot Adler

The "dark" like to destroy for the sole purpose of enjoying people's suffering, and sometimes even in the name of God. But this hive-mind-mentality has been going on for thousands of years. This hive mind is the one who had also overtaken the Goddess temples around the world. They had no respect for the divine feminine or anything sacred. These acts of violence have destroyed cultures and communities across our planet. There has been a war against the sacred since the beginning of time. Spiritual warfare, the kind that we are often too afraid to talk about out loud, is the war against humanity and the feminine.

In my late teens, I moved to America in hopes of a brighter future, one where my unborn children would have access to universal thinking. During my arrival in America in the late '70s, a spiritual revolution was going on, and I found Radhaa's father at the height of the spiritual revolution with a music band named "Prophecy Band." It was almost nearing the end of the Vietnam War, and people were full of passion protesting, standing for freedom, liberty, and justice. The American spirit was strong at that time. There was so much courage and rebellion against the darkness taking place on the planet.

The spiritual community in America was booming, and we attended retreats full of hundreds of people. The teachings of the East were coming into the West, and my husband and I were both reading the Mahabharata when I was pregnant with my Radhaa. We had fallen in love with Goddess Radha and Lord Krsna reading this book. Goddess Radha was unconditionally in love with her beloved--Lord Krsna, and it was a love of unconditional devotion to her beloved. A powerful Sanskrit saying by an ascended Indian Master Shrii Shrii Anandmurtiji, "Shiva-Shakyat Makam Brahma," is a way of saying, "God and Goddess are inseparable, one and the same." Easily referring also to the name and nature of the Goddess/God, and Radhaa was named after Radha and Krishna. It is no wonder why the Goddesses have become Radhaa's ally.

FOREWORD

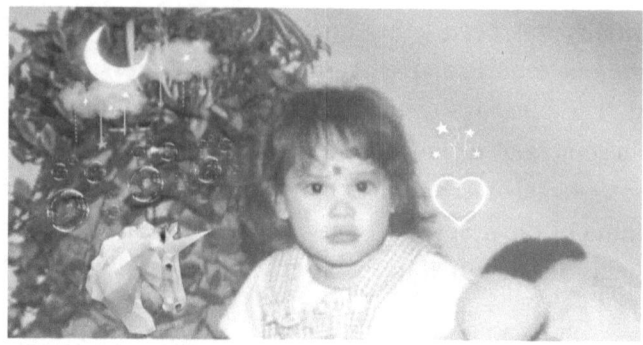

When Radhaa was just a baby (1-year-old), I played with her, adding "bindi" in her 3rd eye, and called her "my little goddess." How funny! This play is almost a futuristic vision and a mystical play we happily delved in as the Goddesses seemingly have approved of.

Radhaa was initiated with the Goddess Energy before she was born, then I took her to Goddess temples and shared her stories of the Goddesses. Through life's traumas and trying to fit in, Radhaa had abandoned the Goddess teachings. And then, a decade ago, I was so thrilled when her Goddesses' visions came flooding back in, calling her back home, and soon her journey back to the Goddesses began. From this, she created Goddess Activations™, her original healing modality.

This book, "Pillars of Light," is a testament to Radhaa's love and devotion to the ancient Goddesses who once walked upon the face of the Earth. Come full circle, Radhaa manifested HERstory as a Goddess activator through the many Goddess Archetypes. She continued to work with women to heal and awaken their inner goddesses. As Radhaa fully expressed her creative genius through Goddess Code Academy, which has become the home for the Divine Feminine, she heard the call again to anchor in the Pillars of Light, Stories of Goddess Activations™'. It was important to call forth these incredible women to gather and represent the Pillars of Light through their Goddess Activations™ initiations. Radhaa saw women worldwide activating their Pillars of Light and creating a new template to help anchor in the Goddess Codes. She kept getting the vision, but it took her a few years to finally manifest it. She offered herself as a Goddess guide to these women who contribute their personal experiences through their writings as Light holders.

Each woman courageously shared their vulnerable stories of pain, suffering, and struggles to clear the old paradigm that held them back as each conquered their rightful place as the feminine truth-tellers. More confidence, self-empowerment, and transformation occur as each unleashes, heals, and clears the old wounded parts of their being.

These women share their inner strength and lessons learned with the world in this book. Their stories embody the feminine resilience and their natural state of evolving into higher consciousness. The up-level of their realizations to position themselves as empowered women in our world through their spiritual understanding is an awakening towards becoming their Pillars of Light. These women are feminine warriors of light, victorious in claiming space as they speak their voices of truth and magic.

May you enjoy this beautiful book created by Radhaa and her magical soul sisters who journey into Goddess Activations™, meeting their Goddess Archetypes in the Pillars of Goddess Light.

Thank you! Salamat Po,
~*Maya The Shaman*

FOREWORD

Saying:

"When women support each other, Miracles happen."

- *Maya the Shaman*

INTRODUCTION
RADHAA NILIA

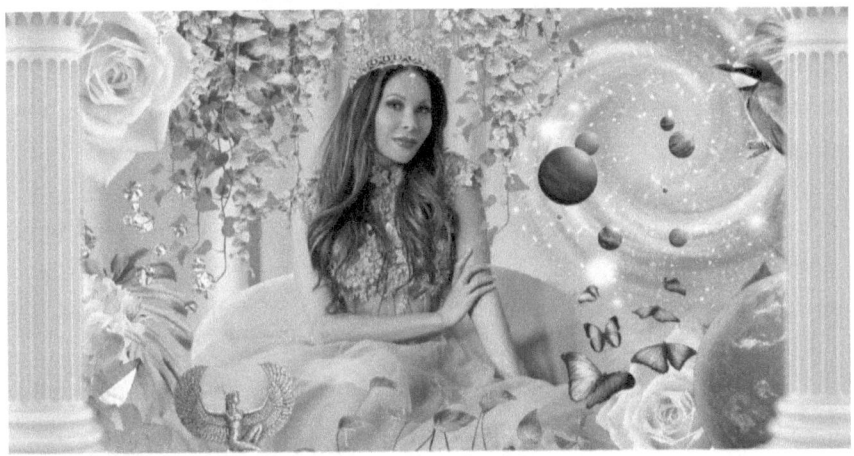

Pillars of Light, Stories of Goddess Activations™, is a feminine fusion of personal stories and Goddess teachings, divine remembrance. I never thought that this was the work I would be doing in a million years. But the Goddess is like that. SHE will take you right off the train tracks to get you back on your Divine Path. She has helped me restore my original Soul blueprints.

My mission is to hold sacred space for the integrity of the

Goddesses and the sacred temple of the Goddess within. The inverted matrix grid has distorted the real essence of a Goddess, given the wrong broadcast message to the collective, and further distorted the Divine Feminine. One reason I decided to trademark my work Goddess Activations™ and Goddess Code™ is to keep the integrity of this sacred work I do. A decade ago, I opened the doors to Goddess Code Academy™, a mystical school for the Divine Feminine. It has become the home of Goddess Activations™ and a temple for the Divine Feminine.

We must start creating temples again, as this is how we anchor the Goddess back into the Earth grid. And it is time on Earth to revive the Goddesses' timeless teachings, pure essence, spiritual presence, feminine healing, and restoration of personal power. The path is complementary to any spiritual practice for your everyday life.

This book offers Goddess Key Codes to help accelerate your inner trust, clarity, and feminine power to your sacred self. Please take each chapter as it's a journey, reading with an open mind and heart, knowing that these courageous women share their personal stories, struggles, and victories through their own lives and with their open hearts and minds in the Goddess Activations™ experience. I honor each woman in each chapter. It's important for me to hold a sacred container in this way. So, if you've picked up this book, it's no coincidence. The Goddess awaits to assist your everyday life, both mystical and practical.

Each Goddess shares her unique gifts, wisdom, and healing energy to Activate the Goddess Code™ within. Goddess Activations™ have brought healings to hundreds of women I have worked with, and now, it is my inner calling to share this work with women worldwide!

Thank you for holding this book in your hands and keeping the Goddess warm in your heart. The SPIRIT of the Goddesses lives in the pages of this book! This journey is one of the greatest remembrances of what the feminine has gone through. May the stories in these pages awaken the Goddess within you.

The Goddesses call you back home to awaken your purpose, your

INTRODUCTION

soul mission to walk your sacred path. You, too, are meant to be the woman of your dreams.

Sisters, it is your time!

RADHAA NILIA

Saying:

"Two thousand years ago, we lived in a world of Gods and Goddesses. Today, we live in a world solely of Gods. Women in most cultures have been stripped of their spiritual power."

~ Dan Brown

CHAPTER 1

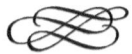

INTRODUCTION TO GODDESS ACTIVATIONS™

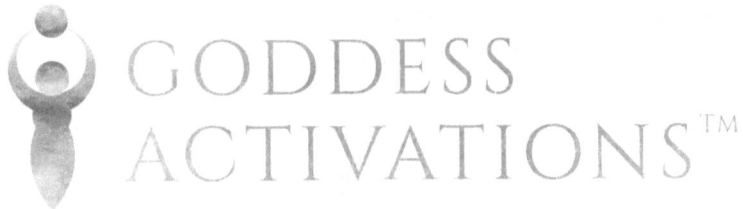

What is **Goddess Activations**™?

Goddess Activations™ is a living light energy transmission, filled with pure Goddess Code™ frequencies. It is different from any other healing modality I've ever experienced. Being a Certified Advanced Teacher and Practitioner of over a dozen healing modalities, I always felt something was missing. So I kept going, more training, more certifications, and six figures later, I was awakened to the missing link.

The Goddess Activations™ is a process of waking up the Goddess Codes™ which currently lie dormant in peoples fields. It's true, we have been tampered on many levels, including our original DNA strands, and now, the time has come to reclaim what truly belongs to us. The question is, are you ready to remember your divinity, innate gifts, inner truth and personal power? This work is a reminder of these sparks that live within you.

Goddess Activations™ is an invitation to fall in love with yourself all over again. Get to know the Goddesses and discover the offerings, guidance, and how you can free yourself from bondage and limitations that hold you back. You will learn that the Goddess energy can spark back up the stagnant energies that need recharging. Goddess Activations™ revives the Goddesses' timeless teachings, pure essence, and spiritual presence, deeply encoded feminine healing and true restoration power.

The false Goddess has inverted the real essence of a Goddess, given the wrong broadcast. The message to the collective further distorted the Divine Feminine. My mission is to restore the integrity of the Goddesses by sharing the stories of Goddess Activations™. Through this sacred work, we balance the scales and bring back the true essence of the authentic Goddesses through Goddess Activations™.

What is a Goddess Code™?

A '**Code**' is a key that unlocks the ability to awaken your dormant Codes within you. Each of the Goddess Codes™ has its unique activations that allow people to create physical manifestations even faster! In true essence, Goddess Activations™ unlocks the Goddess Codes™. It is essential to bring back the original integrity of the "Pillars of Light" through Goddess Activations™.

What is Spinning Goddess™

For Goddess Activations™, I use many Goddess Healing and Clearing tools. One of my favorites is called 'Spinning Goddess™,' Pendulum Healing which we teach at Goddess Code Academy. It's a fun and easy way to clear and reprogram with the Goddess.

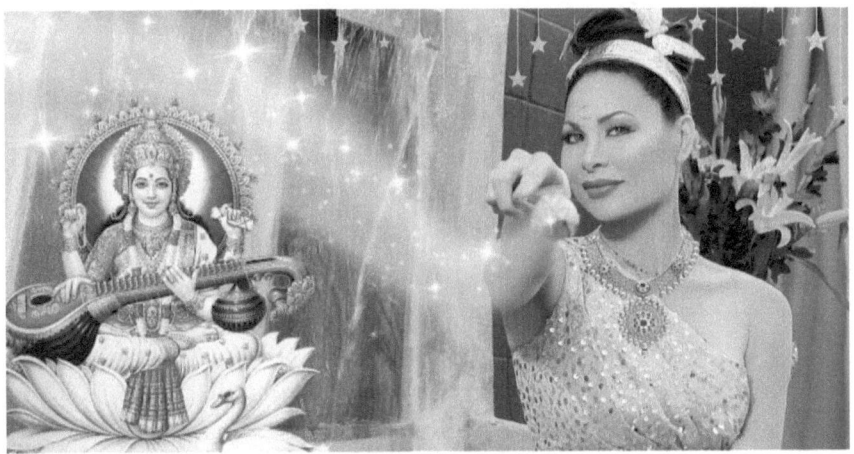

Journey to Your Inner Goddess

In a session, I work with a series of Ancient Goddess Archetypes. We work on a multidimensional level that results in a clearing, healing on a heart and soul level. Everything you need is already inside you, lying dormant. As your Goddess Guide, I help activate the Goddess Code™ inside of you. The Goddess archetype is your superpower. My clients tell me that Goddess Activations™ sessions are unlike anything they have ever experienced before, a blessing from the Divine. Those who are ready to receive this will find a shift, the catalyst that will lead you to the life you are meant to live.

Repatterning with Goddess Activations™

This work deeply reprograms and repatterns you back to your original Soul Blueprint. Clearing away all the distortions and sabotage patterns and beliefs keeping you hostage in a timeline or reality you don't desire. When you step into the sacred initiations through Goddess Activations™, you may experience yourself in a brand new way. Awakened. Sessions are not cookie-cutter but highly intuitive. I tune in with the client's energy 48 hours before a session. When it's time for the session, I do all the intuitive downloads from my 3rd eye as a Goddess seer to my clients. I can see their past lives describe them to clear current issues. No two sessions are ever the same. We decide the Goddess who will be working with you beforehand. If you don't know, I will intuitively connect with the help of your higher self, and together, we choose as this has always been successful.

I use multiple healing methods, being trained and certified in over a dozen healing modalities. During our session, I start with a thirty-minute deep clearing for you. Clearing the space so that we can connect with the Goddess deeper. Then we move into your *Infinite Cosmic Records*™ to meet the Goddess specifically working with you. As we connect with your Goddess, I will receive an influx of information that will be very specific and valuable as a conduit of the Goddess herself. The Goddess will provide her blessings in many areas specific to your needs. And in times, "*the blessings will extend to all other areas of your life that neither of us would even expect.*" At least that's what my clients tell me all the time! You will learn how to access these attributes within you.

The Goddess will inspire, awaken, and elevate your everyday reality. You will restore your confidence as you work with your Goddess and align with her high frequency. It enables you to manifest your desires much easier in the physical world. Goddess Activations™ offer clearing, healing, and cosmic messages. In your session, you can experience the following:

Karmic Clearing
Activate creativity
Activate Abundance
Restore your original blueprint
Remember your Soul's purpose and mission.
Ignite Courage
Elevate your Life
Heal Your Heart Chakra
Help release Soul wounds
Call Back Your Light Essence, and Power
Restore Soul Fragments
Restore self-honor

Restore Inner Trust
Activate Confidence
Awaken your psychic Gifts
Inspire you to move forward in life
Release negative attachments, entities
And cords with ex-partners or lovers

Anchoring Goddess Codes™

It is time to awaken and anchor the Goddess Codes™ into women and humanity. Our Earth grid allows all women to fully recharge to step into our divine feminine power.

It's time to raise the frequency of ourselves and the Planet.

Experience transmissions, where I share each Goddess Code™ before activating the Archetypes individually. If you have worked with me before, you know that this depth and quality of work are priceless. I have been shown that it is important to get these Codes out to as many women as possible who are truly committed and ready to go deep. The Goddess Activations™ is an assignment by the Divine for me to serve humanity.

Embracing Goddess Archetypes

Goddess Activations™ is about activating the Goddess Archetypes. The word "Goddess" is a very sacred word. We know God very well in our society, but the divine feminine aspect has been taken out of texts and scriptures and every aspect of religion. And so now we're feeling the imbalance of that in the world. And it's more important than ever to activate the Goddesses, to bring her back onto planet earth through each woman individually to create that divine feminine archetype and activate the Goddess within.

The word "Goddess" has been misused, like many words nowadays. Goddess Activations™ is very healing as the Goddess is necessary for women to be embodied in their sacred power truly. And we're bringing this sacredness back to the rightful Goddess and bringing sacredness back to ourselves.

I've been working with women one-to-one for over a decade, and I started to feel and see Goddess archetypes drop into the room, literally coming in as energy. And at first, I was a little freaked out, and I was like, what are you doing here?

And as I asked women permission, can I share this with you? I found that it was precisely the Goddess they were working with or felt that energy. And it became this very organic thing where the women were receiving these transmissions from the Goddess. I guess you could say I was a Goddess facilitator, but this became known as Goddess Activations™ because each session activated a dormant Goddess archetype. Once awakened in the feminine, it brought her more healing, peace, joy, and abundance.

After years of working with various women, I realized that the Goddess came through, and it didn't matter what their background or religion. It was this golden thread that wove through, and it brought a sort of healing. It brought a kind of centeredness that they needed in their life. And it wasn't just one Goddess, but multiple Goddesses were coming into my sessions with my clients. Each woman would receive a different Archetypes. Through the years, I started to see patterns and realize how important it is for the Goddess to be part of any woman's healing journey.

HERstory: Remembering

The Goddess is not an intangible concept, idea, or being. The Goddess is real, accessible, and ready to help you on your journey. Whether you envision the Goddess as a living being who comes to assist you in her Archetype, you will benefit as you are called back to your wholeness. Your desire to seek what serves you will be your guide. Through the Goddess Activations™, it is possible to attract the Goddess' essence and activate her power within you. This book is designed to help you connect with Goddess Archetypes through women's stories and experiences. Perhaps you will find something of your own.

How did my work come about? Divine remembrance. My sessions became much more effective when working with the Goddess, and the results were nothing less than miraculous. Over a decade ago, Goddess Activations™ was born through my private healing practice in Hollywood Hills. Goddess Activations™ has been trademarked to protect the integrity of this sacred work.

Goddess Activations™ is an original healing modality I created and the missing link in healing the feminine at the deepest heart and soul level. These Activations are pillars of divine feminine light of pure Shakti Energy.

I've gone through the dark night of my Soul, faced the deepest shadows, and had undertaken many initiations before I was offered this work to women and the world.

> "The very divine primordial Shakti cosmic consciousness moves through the entire Universe. One that we were all originally connected to."

It is time to get aligned with Divine Feminine Consciousness.

> "When you are initiated into your Goddess Activations™, you anchor your Pillar of Light into our Divine Mother Gaia."

As my clients continued to show up to Goddess Code Academy™, I served them with Goddess energies. The Goddess energy is similar to a magic wand or something you may use to eradicate your blockages. She is here to help you spiritually, to help you integrate aspects of yourself that you may have rejected or aspects you may have longed for within yourself.

The value of the Goddess is for us to understand and appreciate HER all aspects of the self in all stages of one's life. Every season of one's life is valuable. Working with the Goddess helps you step into a higher vibration where you can look at the different aspects of how you have lived your life without judgment. The truth is we humans tend to be the harshest critics of ourselves. We don't need more self-judgment. We need to learn to relax into self-love. The Goddess serves as a reminder of our strength, power, or ability to be resilient souls in a human body. Most important of all, please know that you are loved beyond measure. It is something we all need to be reminded of often.

I've turned to the Goddess in my darkest hours, and she is always there with open arms, love, and acceptance. If you can learn to appreciate all the Goddess aspects within yourself, your life experience will expand exponentially. It's like being an artist with only charcoal to work with, and discovering a whole spectrum of colors available to paint with is like getting to know the Goddesses. The expression will be far richer with infinite possibilities. It is how I experienced Goddess Activations™ when this powerful "Shakti Energy" all started to come through.

My experiences have provided me the strength to move forward with the quest for a deeper meaning in life. In doing so, my process kept me assisting others through the Goddess Activations™. Each Goddess would bring something new, and I felt I was getting fast-tracked in my Goddess essence, energy, and studies in real-time with each Goddess.

First and foremost for women, but not limited to just women. Men can learn from the feminine experience as well, and they can learn how to honor and respect women. As I first processed information, I embodied my work as a Goddess Guide and found many women clients gravitated towards me, eager to make their journey to the Goddess. It has been an honor to hold a sacred space for their healing and transformations.

During a Goddess download, I allowed the Goddesses to bring whatever gifts of healing we needed. For HER, gifts can flow through you without expectations. These gifts never come by way of assumptions or demands, and it is shared with you by a powerful exchange of trust and openness that occurs.

As I witnessed women awaken to the Goddess within, it was as if a whole new reality opened up for them as it had for me. They found a safe place to be supported and expanded into many layers of their wholeness, which is the beginning of the Pillars of Light within Goddess Activations™.

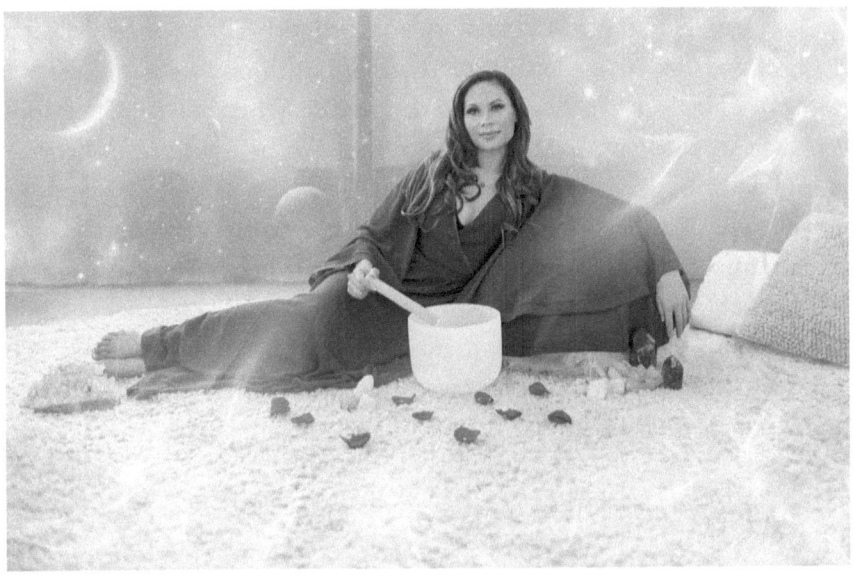

"*Pillars of Light, Stories of Goddess Activations™ was born and continues to unfold and reveal new truths.*"

The gifts of the Goddesses are blessings and rewards that come only through authenticity, dedication, and sincerity from my clients. When you experience Goddess Activations™, you will also discover that they are the "living truth and the living light codes." That is why it is vital to understand the gateways to the Goddesses through the Pillars of Light, Goddess Activations™.

I have seen my clients shift and do incredible things from the experience of Goddess Activations™. These changes include more self-confidence, personal fulfillment, enigmatic presence, a sense of pride in sharing who she is, and the ability to manifest what she wants in life.

The women who journeyed with the Goddess grew exponentially in a very short period! Some have even found the love of their life after learning to love themselves deeply.

"Coming to Earth as a human is one of the most challenging tasks we could ever encounter as soul beings."

We are so much more than this experience. Yet, we become so defined and imprisoned in our own making through the beliefs we take on. Our lives are created and destroyed by our beliefs. Therefore we must be discerning on what we commit to believing in to be true to ourselves.

It's time for the Goddess energy to reign on Earth again through the feminine embodiment of a living woman. I now share with others these teachings through the institute I founded called "Goddess Code Academy™." I've discovered that connecting women back to the Goddesses has helped my clients heal their deepest wounds. Wounds that were very hard to reach deep inside of them.

" The fear of speaking her truth or being who she is truly meant to be has caused a silent pain and suffering for so many women."

We all need a sacred space to heal the dark wounds that have held us hostage in the deepest recesses of our being. The freedom to speak one's truth and express oneself is vital in living one's life. Realizing this unbearable need for truth, women seek answers. Many women these days are willing to do the deep healing work required towards their liberation.

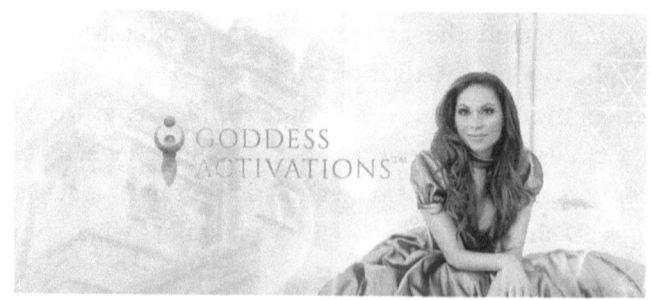

CHAPTER 2

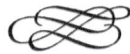

PERSONAL STORIES OF GODDESS ACTIVATIONS™

Radhaa Nilia

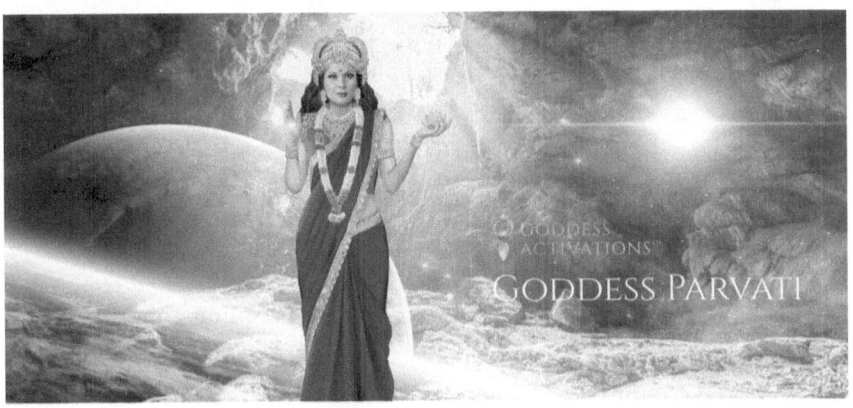

Salutations To The Goddess

"I offer salutations to the Goddess: The infinite Creatrix of the Universe. The Feminine aspect of God, the giver of all life." - **Radhaa**

The Dali Lama said, "*The World will be saved by the Western Woman.*" I believe that too, and I believe in the power of the divine feminine. As you can see, the healthy, grounded, fierce, loving, fully self-expressed wild woman, empowered with divine feminine leadership is needed now more than ever on Earth. Feminine energy has been intentionally distorted in our world for so long. In ancient times there were Goddess Priestess temples that could be found everywhere.

But in this modern time, we find that most ancient Goddess temples have been destroyed, along with the teachings and the initiations that went with them. The imbalance on our Planet has caused chaos and confusion due to the dark takeover. This has disturbed the hearts and minds of women and men, individually and collectively at large. It is time to bring healing, balance, and sacred remembrance with the divine feminine. It is time to restore the sacred temple of the Goddess within. Women who walk through these Pillars of Light receive soul medicine through Goddess Activations™. It is time to bring forward Goddess Activations™.

The following pages contain several stories I am sharing with you about my past life to the present. Through diving into my past, so many pieces of the puzzle came along with the initiations I had to walk through before presenting this work. The path of the Goddess is not always easy. Those who feel the call have probably struggled in so many ways in this life and past lives. Always coming up against the dark controllers, offending for simply existing.

Yet here we all are, and we must take every experience encoded in our DNA and transmute it as the Alchemist. We must remember our sacred selves. And this is what the Goddess has taught me. She's been relentless in training me lifetimes upon lifetimes, to be sharing this work at this level. I had to come to terms with healing and forgiveness for my past experiences, such as stories you are about to read in the next pages, entitled: "Trampled Temples," "Past Burning Into The Present," and "Stepping Into The Sisterhood."

TRAMPLED TEMPLES

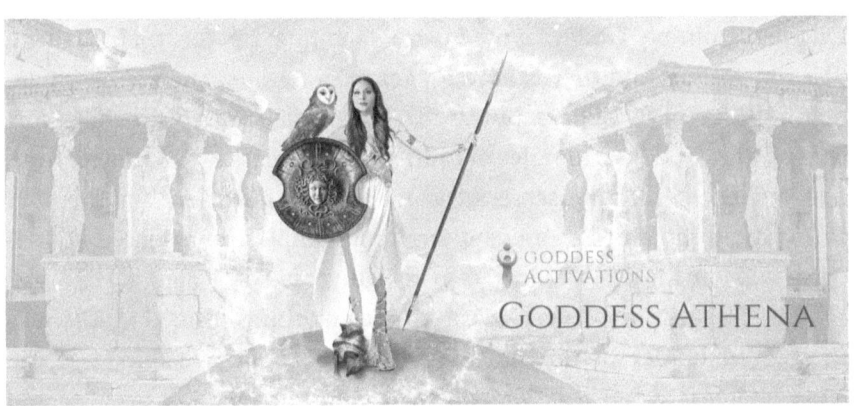

There has been historical evidence of an unearthed matriarchal society that shows numerous artifacts, sculptures, paintings, and existing matrilineal societies scattered around the globe. And even in my journey through past life regressions, I was brought back to a time where I worked in one of the sacred temples as a Priestess. The Goddess energy reigned on Earth from 30,000 BCE to 2000 CE. I was part of the Goddess temples in Europe, specifically Greece. Women worked together in harmony, peace, and beauty. It was at that time when the patriarchy infiltrated our temples. Those who wanted to rule, take over, and dominate the sacred space. There was no room for the feminine. Their armies came to our temples to destroy us, and we ran for our lives.

It's been said that 600 million women were burnt as witches, and the patriarchy of the ancient past destroyed their temples. It was the most undiscussed, undocumented yet most destructive genocides on Planet Earth. I find it interesting Churches have taken over many of the Goddess sites for the purpose of tapping into the feminine womb energy that was placed before. And now, it's time to resurrect the truth.

This remembrance of the divine feminine persecution is an awakening in the psyche of modern women. It is no longer a secret. The once Goddess Temples became the ruthless massacre grounds of the Divine Feminine. Today, women are standing up for their rightful place in society, and they can no longer tolerate the abuse. Women are not fighting with bullets but by their courageous spirits in resurrecting the Goddess temples within. The Goddess was deleted from our awareness for thousands of years as we knew her, but the soul scars would remain. The ancient feminine temples represented knowledge, wisdom, and power in this great Universe.

The Goddess was everywhere in ancient times. The Goddess was the sacred holder of feminine love, devotion and wisdom, but the story changed when this version of the patriarchy took over. Sacred Goddesses were deleted from history and our very consciousness. This toxic takeover came with the arrogant attitude, "*We know better.*"

As you can see around the World at this time, the stronghold of the patriarchy is still trying to control our every breath literally and in reality. As this battle for control heightens and can be felt by all, it is true that these controllers and this old paradigm is dying as we reclaim our hearts, minds, bodies, and wombs.

As we awaken the Goddess within, we are anchoring the Goddess back on Earth. The time is coming for us to share stories and open up the pathways to healing. But before we can do that, we must first take responsibility for our bleeding wounds and step into our temple of healing and transformation. We start to integrate and embody the fullness that we truly are through the Goddess Archetypes and Activations.

These memories I'm sharing in this chapter represented a time of terror for me where I felt utterly powerless. These themes of powerlessness played out in many of my past and presented lifetimes over and over again. Because of these Soul trauma experiences, I had become fearful of taking ownership of possessing my power. And in this life, although I was pushed down, suppressed, and told to shut up by an abusive caretaker, I have found that through exploring ways of facing my fears and using my voice by immersing myself in my artistic endeavors, I knew I had to break free of the invisible grip that had been around my neck.

So, to face these excruciating fears, I decided to enroll in a prestigious acting school in Hollywood. I chose this school with the acclaimed teacher, Howard Fine, because I knew it would push me out of my comfort zone and step right up into using my voice.

I would shake in my seat as my scenes approached. Shivering like a leaf in the wind. But when they called my name, I would take a deep breath, the complete wreck of nerves and praying my voice would indeed come through. I was brave because otherwise, I wanted to run out the doors and straight to the bathroom to vomit from the sickness of being in front of everyone. Even though many of these people had become my dear friends and I so admired and adored them, I did not feel safe taking up space since most of my childhood was huddled in a room trying to stay small, to stay clear of an abuser, whom, if I crossed paths, would go on a tirade of screams, insults, and destroy my healthy sense of self. It was so much safer to hide. So I forced myself into this precarious position of being on stage to be seen.

I was up to do a big scene in front of my acting class. Walking up to the stage, it was huge and tall. My legs were shaking. My character was enraged after being betrayed, and I surely have felt that way many times over in my own life. I had a rage that brewed deep in my belly. I tapped into it. It was a rumble, a volcano, a fire. I could feel it. Oh, it started so well, but then I couldn't climax to the fullness of my furry. All the times I had been shoved down, told to shut up, suppressed, it was all there, but I was blocked. When it came time for me to scream, my voice betrayed me. The scream was stuck in my throat, burning, burning, burning. Hot tears filled my eyes. Why the f--k couldn't I scream?

Where was she, my inner Kali that I had felt years and years like a madwoman, a demon slayer after these abuses? The audience was silent, and I knew they were all praying for me. The tension in the studio was high. My acting partner was pissed I had failed her. I was startled when Howard Fine screamed at me at the top of his lungs, "Radhaa, own your POWER!" That shook me to the core. I could not express or unleash this primal rage and power required in this particular scene. I was frozen at the moment, but he successfully awakened something deep and dormant inside of me. Although I burned with humiliation and defeat, I also felt the raw truth in his words.

The fear of being persecuted or punished for speaking up, taking up space, sharing the truth has caused silent pain and suffering for me at that moment. And later on, my journey to find my silent screams, my voice, I came to understand this grief that lives silently in so many women. It wasn't an acting class I needed, but a sacred space to heal the deepest and darkest of wounds that have held me hostage in the recesses of my being.

Realizing this unbearable need for the freedom to speak my truth and express myself was as vital as breathing air. I was dying a slow death. I continued taking classes and later found Comedy to speak harsh and unbearable truths in a way that people could laugh at. I enjoyed the darkness of Comedy. You didn't have to scream and cry on stage, you could stand there and deliver the most f-up shit, and people would sit and laugh at it. It lifted some pressure off my chest, and I even got invited to perform at the Comedy Store. I enjoyed the laughs so much that at least someone could laugh at my misery.

Comedy is truly sadistic, and somehow it soothed my soul at the time. I had been humiliated a lot as a child, brought into a room full of adults who would talk badly about me, and I would stand there completely frozen, and I swallowed it all. It was their unprocessed emotions, anger, pain, fear, trauma. I was the one who ate others' emotions for them. There was nowhere to run. Comedy was a lot like that, except I was the one who was saying all of these things. And in a way, it was taking my power back. If anyone is going to talk shit about me, it's going to be me. Weirdly, I felt part of myself returning from doing Comedy. I loved and hated it. The nights I bombed, and I did, the humiliation appeared all over again. The nights that I killed it, I felt like I was on top of the World. My inner child was gleaming. Yet, I kept having a nagging feeling that there was something deeper I needed to explore. It was healing I desired, healing I needed.

And later, when I went deeper into my healing, I understood what my acting teacher was talking about. My fear of my power had haunted me my whole life.

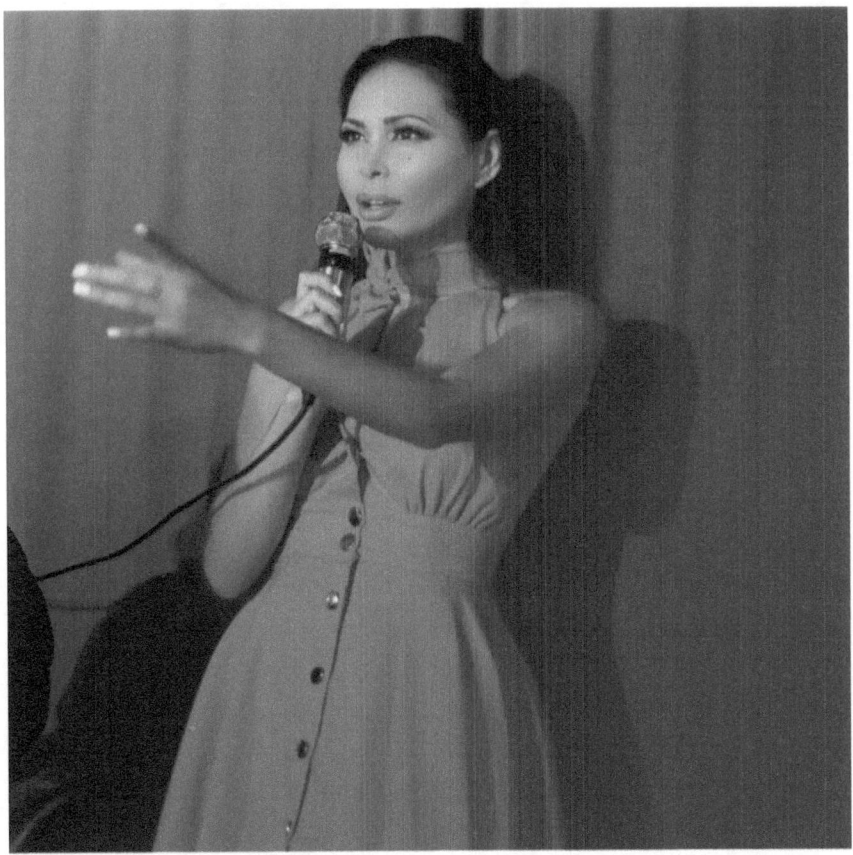

Throughout my life, I was much more comfortable giving my power away than taking ownership of it. Yet another part of me was courageous and ready to try something daring and new. My only motivation was to find my pieces and put them back together again.

The Goddess has helped me in understanding that there are indeed many inner Archetypes, and not just the pretty and pleasing ones. The Goddess goes beyond what society thinks is pleasing. The Goddess has many faces, and many of them are not the ones people want to see, in HER or themselves.

If my inner Goddess is raging, there is no doubt there's a good reason for it. If I need to shout at the top of rooftops to share a message that must be heard, I certainly will. If I feel a passion for a project, I must do it without a doubt.

A woman who walks this path may not be perfect, but she is not always going to be just pretty and sweet. According to every situation, a true woman will be the way she needs to be. I made a promise to the Goddess to no longer live as a people pleaser. Rather, I promise to be true to the voice of my Soul, not always easy, but a lifelong commitment.

I breathed deeply into this understanding, *"A safe haven, A home, A temple."* I didn't have to be perfect to be loved. I didn't have to prove my worth, entertain or please others. I was embraced by the Goddesses for who I am, for simply being a child of the Divine.

The Goddess is the giver of true integration. Embracing all aspects of my being is liberating. It has given me so much hope, freedom, and healing, that I humbly bowed to the Goddess in all her faces.

The many feminine Archetypes have assisted me on my journey. When She led me to step into holistic healing as a practitioner and later to create the Goddess Activations™ method, I followed it's every step of the way. I thank the Goddesses, for being my guiding light, even into the ancient past of trampled temples where she guided me to break these old curses. It was finally time to set me free.

Embracing ALL sides. The Goddess allowed me to DARE to love all sides of myself, including the rageful one, the hurt, the angry, the bitch, the fraught, the villain, the victim, the sensual, the playful, the lover, mystic, friend, caretaker, nurturer, healer, empath, creatrix, warrior, etc. Since it's *so* easy to accept the lovable Archetypes, it is equally important to integrate the shadow aspects that we all embody, those which are not pretty, not pleasing, not perfect, such as the outcast, the reject, because the Goddess embodies everything, including the supernatural.

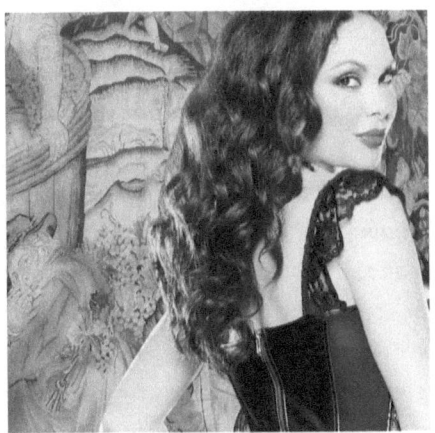

Breaking the Curse

"I've been cursed a thousand times,
Not just in this life but a hundred others.
By friends, by lovers, others who called me names,
Outcast, Witch, Whore, and Priestess.
I've run for my life so many times, but not anymore.
Today I stand where I am.
I look the perpetrator in the eyes.
What more can you possibly take from me,
That you've not already taken before?
My dignity, my family, my body, my life.
Though you have succeeded many times over,
You still come back for more and more and more.
Let me ask you this dear one:
What kind of love do you need?
What kind of hunger do you have?
What kind of thirst do you feel?
How may I serve you?
How may I love you?
How may I forgive you?
How may I hold you close to my breasts?
Though I've had my chest cut wide open,

Yet, healing still flows from my heart.
Don't you see, love?
Your savage ways only hurt yourself.
With every curse, you curse yourself.
Every sword you swing cuts you deeply.
Your blinding pain is a call for help from the Divine.
What you don't understand is that the Divine is within you.
Take time to nurture your heart that feels insatiable.
You will never be satisfied by drinking the life force of another.
Instead, you will be left with a greater thirst than before.
I may have been killed a thousand different ways,
A thousand different times, I never truly died.
For here I stand before you,
Here to remind you.
You deserve to know love.
You deserve to know your own love."
~Radhaa

PAST BURNS INTO THE PRESENT

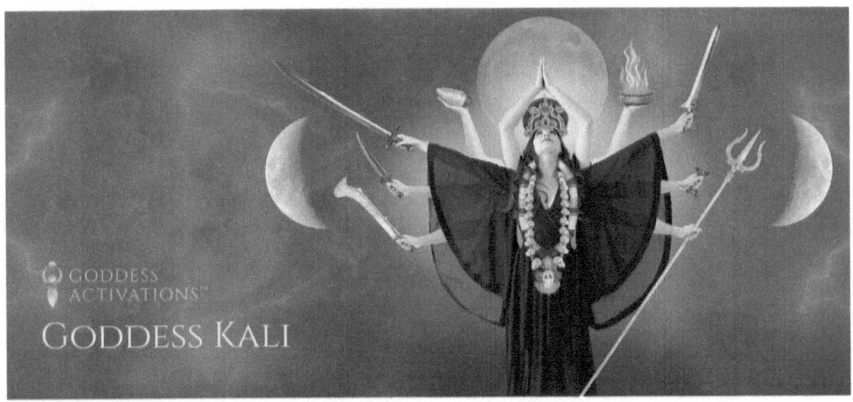

*I*n another past life regression with Goddess Activations™, I went into the fire of my demise. The Betrayal of the Feminine in New England, and I had been an apprentice under a male alchemist. It was a secretive mentorship where I had learned to be an alchemist myself. I felt I had learned everything from my mentor and no longer needed his guidance. We still had a friendship, and I was very grateful for his mentorship. I thought all was well. I was happily married with a child.

My husband was too busy to know about my alchemical abilities because I kept up the image of an ordinary life that mostly included tending to the typical duties of tending home and family. Little did I know my mentor was secretly seething with resentment. I had come into my own, remembering my abilities from other lifetimes; I did not need to be dependent anymore. He went to the authorities and reported me as a witch. I was dragged from my family home and was put into jail until it was time for my trial.

In my regression, I saw myself on the stand. I was wearing an outfit of a large skirt with a petticoat and collar that was so uncomfortable. My throat felt so restricted, and I recalled feeling like I couldn't breathe. There were what seemed like hundreds of angry men filling the courthouse, some wearing funny wigs and short weird pants. I was frozen in fear.

They demanded that I speak or defend myself, and I could do neither. It went on for far too long as the court read off a list of all the sins I had allegedly committed. "Fabricated lies," I recalled in my regression, thinking that there is no way out, no escape, no defending myself, and no winning. These kinds of trials were relatively new at the time, but there was such a fever around this calling-out of witches that these men were almost foaming at the mouth to see me persecuted.

I looked out at the audience and saw my mentor. He was smug, and he had achieved what he wanted and would never be threatened by me again. We both knew my fate. The voices blended into a murmur. I wondered how it would feel about dying. I was helpless and hopeless. I looked out at my husband, who was as helpless as I was, and I regretted ever beginning my work with this mentor.

Our relationship started as acquaintances at the local market. I had seen him a few times at the outdoor market, more like hanging out, and we smiled in passing. One day he casually chatted with me about how I came to be here in this town and asked how I liked living here. He gained my Trust with his offer of easy friendship, which was welcome to me as a newcomer.

One day, he said he wanted to show me something. He lived right around the corner, and I didn't think much of it, so I stopped by after shopping at the market. He wanted to read me something, a book of herbs used medicinally. When he did, something lit up inside of me. It was an energy of new excitement. He saw my spark and asked if I wanted to learn more. But of course, I did. And that is how this mentorship began. We made holistic medicine from herbs. I had a thing with nature, and it came naturally to me. I could configure plant chemistry based on my intuition rather than what was instructed in the books. At first, he was delighted that he could get so much out of me.

There was a black market for such things, and he sold them to make his living. I didn't care for the money, nor did I ask him for payment in exchange for my labor. I was more intrigued by how these remedies could help people. It was exciting to think I had such a skill that was out of the ordinary. I began to spend more time creating concoctions for him, but then it began to take a toll on my household and my child.

I needed to be at home much more than I had been. So I told my mentor, "Thank you, but I will not be able to work any longer on these concoctions." He seemed to understand, and we went our separate ways. I saw him at the market a few weeks later, and he begged me to please help him with some orders. I told him I could not, but I could make them at my own home to be with my child and meet him at the market the following week. He asked me to make the largest batch I could and that it would be the last time he would ask for such a favor.

That day, I took home extra herbs and bottles that would be needed for this task. I did as I said I would, and the following week I brought as much as I could in the form of tinctures.

I told him that would be the last time I could help him and that I had a few more bottles at home should he need them. He smiled and said he understood. I thanked him for showing me how to create home remedies, and I would be able to help my family now when I'm needed. We went our separate ways again. Soon after, I was arrested in my home. The authorities said someone had reported that I was brewing witch potions and casting spells at my home.

I instantly knew who had reported me, yet I could not understand why. Had I not helped this man and asked for nothing in return, I would not be crucified. Had I not paid my debt off to him by creating concoctions for him to sell for introducing me to the book that showed me how to use herbs? In the courtroom, he looked very calm amongst the chaos. They brought the tinctures to the stand as a form of evidence. They asked me where I had learned such witchery and what was I planning to do with these tinctures? Who was I planning on poisoning?

I told them that they were made of herbs and not dangerous at all. My words were dismissed and scoffed at. I glanced at my mentor. He had a smirk on his face. I was confused. Then the judgment came that I was pronounced an evil witch who would pay for the sins I had been accused of. I was shocked and numbed. I looked out at the sea of men's faces where there was a feeling of excitement, of winning; they were celebrating my execution!

The next thing I knew, I was tied to a stake with my arms behind my back, my ankles and legs tightly bound to a thick wooden pole. My feet were on top of a pile of sticks and wood that would serve as fuel for my fire. By having the fire start at my feet, I would endure a slow, searing, and painful death. My face would be the last to be seen in flames so everyone could see my dying expression.

In my session, I recalled the flames at my feet burning so strong my body went into shock, blocking the severity of the pain. All I saw was a sea of eyes staring at me, and no one came forward to defend me. My husband was on his knees crying before me, not daring to look at me. I was the entertainment for the sadistic ritual of killing witches. The crackle of the sticks burning and the smell of my flesh being cooked alive served to excite the apathetic audience. I could not even scream, and I could only surrender to my impending death, wishing it to be swifter than it was.

I felt death was too slow, and in my pain-wracked agony, I prayed for a quick death. The last thing I saw in the corner of the crowd was my mentor, standing tall, standing still, just staring at me. I looked into his cold eyes before I departed from my life, wondering why.

Yet, here I am again, reborn into another lifetime. These experiences and lifetimes have served me well. I am here to reclaim Divine Feminine energy with a ferocious fire in my heart. I came for this, and I desire to reignite the Souls who have been injured throughout the dark times. It's time to rebirth these Codes, to ignite that inner fire of truth, wisdom, and knowing. The Goddess must be here on Earth, and the longer the absence of HER energy not anchored within the feminine, the more imbalanced the World shall be.

STEPPING INTO SISTERHOOD

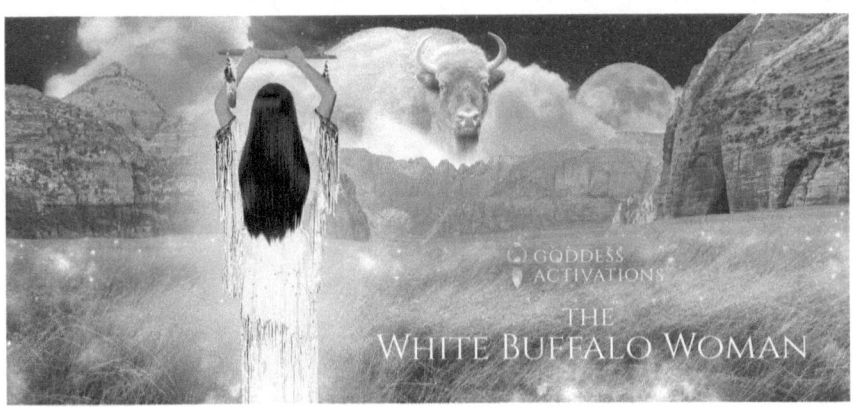

*A*s each woman activates her own healing and empowerment, she can honor her sisters without feeling competitive or pushing other down.

Since I was a child, I've been at the receiving end of women's projections, including hate and jealousy. It's an exhausting cycle that has broken my heart thousand times over. I knew I had to get to the root of why women are cruel to themselves and each other. In my understanding, women have been taught not to love themselves. Society has bred an environment of competition and unnecessary rivalry amongst women. The competition was one of the patriarchy's realm. It weakens the bond within ourselves and with others. By walking the way of The Goddess Code™ and its Activations™, we can learn to uplift and empower ourselves with each other. Let us heal together, as sisters in humanity.

Saying:

"The Goddess has never been lost. It is just that some of us have forgotten how to find her."

~ Patricia Monaghan

ABOUT RADHAA NILIA

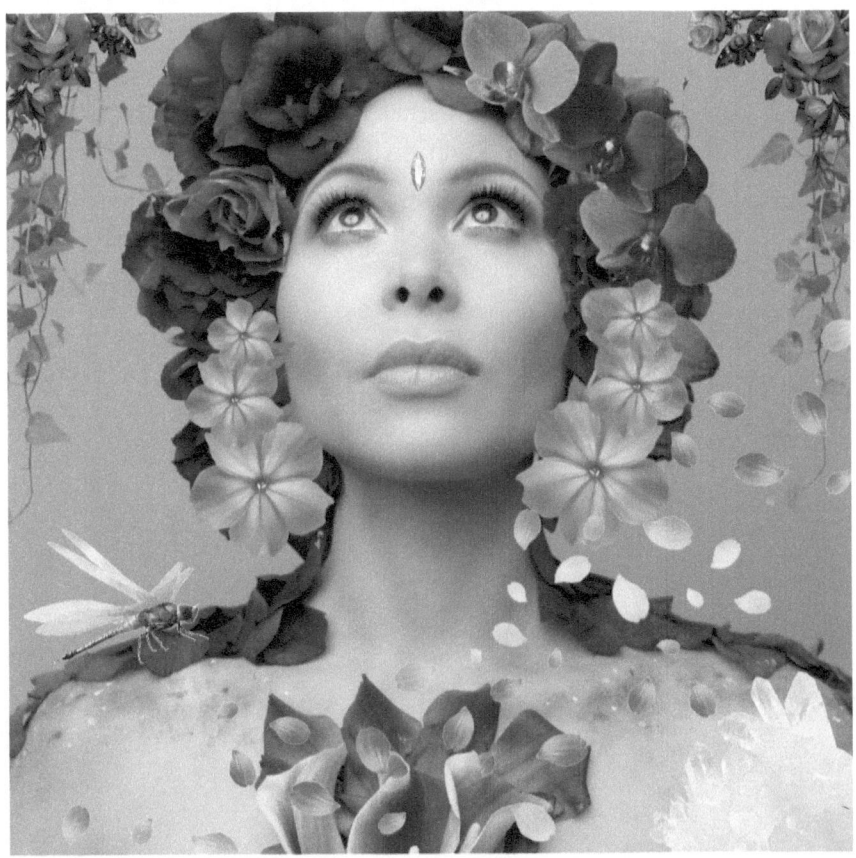

Radhaa Nilia is a multimedia artist, coach, and teacher. Radhaa is the curator and author of the Awakening Starseeds book series. She loves bringing together voices around the world to share their stories.

Radhaa works with women to activate their inner Goddess, heal their heart wounds and souls to find their higher purpose at Goddess Code Academy™, A mystical school for the divine feminine where she provides certification programs and teaches her original healing modality called Goddess Activations™: https://radhaanilia.net/goddess-activations/

Additionally, Radhaa is the founder of Radhaa Publishing House and a contributing writer for various online magazines such a Huffington Post, Elephant Journal, Splash Magazine and continues to Curate collaborative books for Authors voices to shine through. Find out more @ www.RadhaaPublishingHouse.com

To find Radhaa go to:
www.RadhaaNilia.net

CHAPTER 3

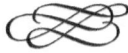

PELE GODDESS ACTIVATIONS™

Hilda Zamora

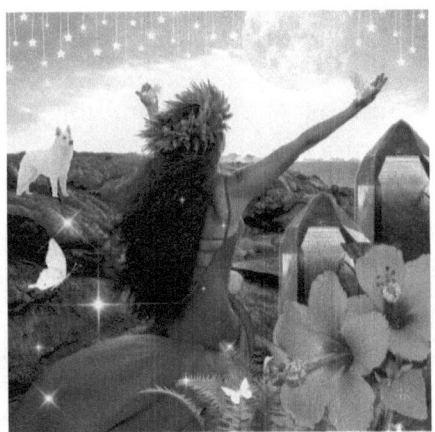

I remember that day as if it were yesterday. It was a nice, warm, sunny day. One of my uncles came to visit. Being her usual, hospitable self, my mom fed him with whatever little we had while they talked for a bit. On that very day, I made a big fuss about wanting to meet my godmother – who happened to be this uncle's daughter-in-law as well. I always enjoyed spending time with her, and on that particular day, I wanted to see her.

Her house was a street over. Since I was only five years old at the time, my mom obviously wouldn't let me go by myself. At the same time, she couldn't take me herself because she was busy with some household chores. My uncle pitched in since he was going to walk over there anyway. He suggested that he'd take me. My mom, of course, agreed. I didn't have any qualms either; I trusted him. All of my elders were nice – or so I thought.

I waved to my mom as we walked out. We walked along the route like usual till he took a detour. Because I've walked down the path to her house countless times, I asked him why we didn't go from where we usually did, to which he replied that he was taking me through a "shortcut." I didn't think twice about it and followed along.

We eventually came across this house under construction. It had no roofs or rooms. It only had four walls and a small opening in one of them, serving as a window. It didn't seem like anyone had lived there in a long time – there were weeds, and the floor was covered in dust. As we stood by the door, I was hesitant to go inside – why would he take me here? My uncle reassured me and told me it was perfectly fine. The respect and trust ingrained in our minds for our elders made me stop questioning him, and I went inside.

I was five years old. Five. Years. Old. This man undressed me and molested me. A five-year-old girl was robbed of her innocence. In situations like these, time seems to slow down. I was so young; I couldn't even comprehend what was happening. All I knew was that whatever this was, it was wrong – it should not be happening. I was traumatized and completely paralyzed. I couldn't scream for help or do anything. I lay there, comatose. In those handfuls of minutes, my trust in my elders was completely shattered.

As my torment continued, I turned my head toward the window, peering outside, hoping, praying that someone would come to my aid. As luck would have it, an aunt, who must have heard my whimpers, came up to the window and saw us. She yelled out, asking what my uncle was doing to me – to which he told her to get lost. Begrudgingly, that's what she did. My would-be savior, who could have helped end the torment, left. She looked me right in the eyes and saw what exactly he was doing to me, but she still left. She didn't even call for help, nothing; she just left me there to suffer.

The human brain is an enigma. I remember every detail of this tragedy, yet nothing after it. I draw a blank. I don't know what happened, where I went, who found me. All I remember are vague recollections, my mom carrying me back home, sobbing as she did. I still couldn't process what happened; all I knew was that whatever did happen was terrible.

My mom took me back home. My clothes at the time were drenched. I was so young, so innocent, my only concern at that moment was that my mom would scold me – thinking I peed myself. I kept telling her that I didn't. She wouldn't stop kissing and hugging me, profusely apologizing. My mom took off all of my clothes and put them in a pile outside the house – where she burnt them. Many women from my family gathered around Pretty soon, crying in unison as they hugged and kissed me. As touched as I was by their support, I was mostly disappointed. Instead of doing something about it, they chose to hide it from the men in the village. They kept on saying how this was about "protecting me," which was hypocritical. The worst already happened. I already felt like a broken, soulless shell of a person.

I couldn't even properly comprehend what exactly had happened, yet I knew, whatever it was, it was unjust. As the days passed after this incident, I felt like no one stood up for me. My mom never reported him to the authorities, either. Despite her knowing who he was – she did nothing. Perhaps this was because we had nothing; we were nobodies. She must have been scared of the ramifications this would have had. The justice system in Mexico works a lot differently than in America. In Mexico, you would need to buy justice to get justice.

Throughout my formative years, I constantly thought about how there could be more innocent girls who had to endure that monster's wrath. This single traumatic event lit a fire in me, the fire of justice. I wanted to be the voice of the people who couldn't speak up for themselves, the voice of people who needed justice and couldn't get it, the voice Hilda so desperately needed but never got.

I have been working with Radhaa to cure this trauma for many years. When Radhaa offered me the opportunity to represent Goddess Pele and learned about her, I could not bear the emotional turmoil that arose from my soul. I learned Goddess Pele is the Goddess of passion, sensuality, and wildness. She represents the lower chakra energies (i.e., root and sacral), and she is both feared and revered by the Hawaiian people. To me, Pele represents the pure feminine and primal mystery as she is both creator and destroyer. I immediately identified with Goddess Pele's power and purpose.

To date, it is hard to let go of my traumatic experience. Radhaa has helped me release this pain, anger, and resentment throughout the years through her unique Goddess Activations™ Codes. Through the Goddess Activations™ Codes, she has taught me to accept, love, and respect myself. She has also taught me how to notice my awareness of who I am.

During my Goddess Activations™ Session with Goddess Pele, she gave me a hibiscus flower to represent her embodying me. She worked on healing my throat chakra and clearing my blocks. You see, although my perpetrator has been dead for over 15 years now, the wounds persist. I have hated myself for the longest time, without even realizing why. Throughout this time, I have felt that justice was not rendered. I have felt that I was prevented from speaking my truth for so many years. No wonder Goddess Pele first focused on my throat chakra, which is responsible for communication, self-expression, and the ability to speak your truth.

Secondly, Goddess Pele focused on my root chakra. The root chakra corresponds to the earth element and the roots we've planted, how strong they are, how deep they are, and how supportive they are. It consists of whatever grounds you for stability in your life. That includes basic needs like food, water, shelter, safety, and emotional needs like letting go of fear and anxiety. When in balance, we feel grounded and safe. When out of balance, we feel anxious, insecure, and vulnerable. I have experienced scarcity on every level throughout my life, not to mention the sense of insecurity and vulnerability that such trauma has left engraved in my body.

After Goddess Pele spoke through Radhaa, I felt her fire within me and a sense of security and protection I had not felt before. I understand that I can only bring the five-year-old me justice by being the voice of good for those who need it. I never want to be that vulnerable girl in that run-down house ever again. Justice and integrity have always been core values for me. For me, it's not just about winning the case as an attorney; it's about providing justice to those who need it. Goddess Pele helps me find the spark in myself that at times it is so easy to lose sight of, for not only my trauma but also the line of work I have as a family law practitioner and defense attorney.

It is a daily battle for me; do I win, or do I lose? Goddess Pele, through Radhaa, helped me resolve my inner knowing: it motivates me, brings in the spark inside me, and makes me feel powerful and in control of my feelings and past beliefs.

If you've been in my place, know; you learn to live with the pain. Invoke the Goddess Pele's energy through the use of crystals and gemstones to include lava stone and obsidian as well as the elemental energy of fire. Use it as fuel for your dreams, become the person you've always wanted to be. Most importantly, never be afraid to do or say the right things; be the voice of justice for the unfortunate, help people the best you can, and no matter how terrible things get, accept life the way it is, push yourself off the ground, wipe the dirt, and move on. It won't be easy, but it is the only way forward.

Remember, you are not thrown in the fire. You are the fire!

Saying:

"A queen keeps a court that is spoken about. A Goddess keeps a court that is never forgotten."

~ Nalini Singh

HILDA ZAMORA

~ CONTRIBUTING WRITER ~

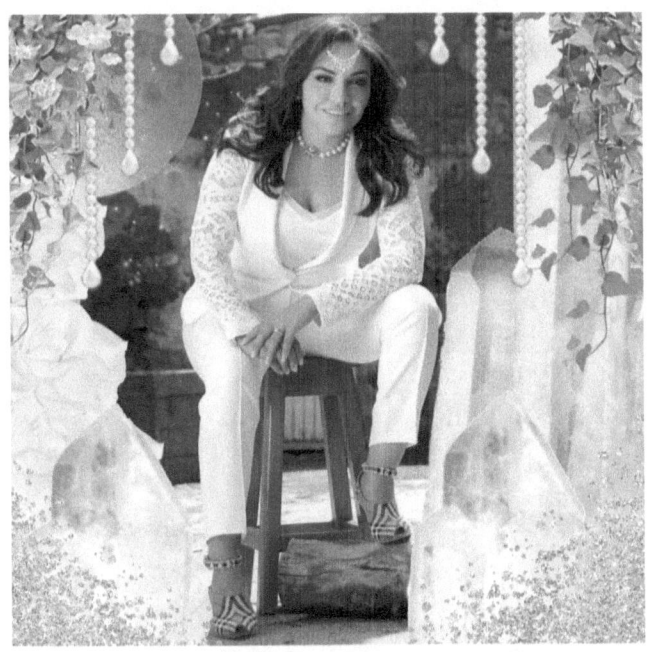

Hilda Zamora is an attorney, author, and speaker in feminine empowerment. As a woman that has overcome much adversity, Hilda is a woman who refuses to be defeated. She uses her pain to fuel her inner-fire, never giving up even when she feels she could not keep going. Hilda wishes to share her experience and help other women who may feel broken inside, unworthy of a better life, tired, or hopeless due to current circumstances in their life.

To connect or reserve her attendance at a women's retreat or be a speaker, feel free to contact her via email at:
   Hello@empoweredboss.co

CHAPTER 4

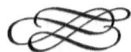

APHRODITE GODDESS ACTIVATIONS™

Danielle Schreck

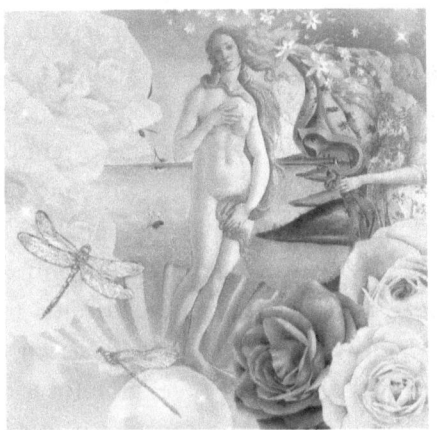

*E*very moment leading up to now has brought me to the experience of this beautiful Goddess Activations™. I am so thankful to our Creator that I connected to Radhaa through the organic series of synchronicities leading to this Activation. Since I can remember, it felt like I was always being guided, supported, and led towards embracing my inner feminine power.

I have always been a girly girl, and before my father remarried, I was a bit of a "Daddy's Girl." Prior to my parent's divorce, the attention was solely on me as an only child. I somehow subconsciously transferred the tentativeness of my fathers babying me into a belief I couldn't do things myself which caused a feeling of disempowerment as I grew. Somehow, it gave me a feeling of being cared for and not trusting I could do things myself. That's where I learned my sense of inner power was outside of me and through someone else, which led me to not trusting myself confidently, and this is the foundation from my perspective that taught me one of the greatest lessons as an Adult.

My father was the first to remarry and received custody of me shortly after their divorce. That was hard on my mother and caused a lot of strain on our relationship over the years. From then on, I spent the next twelve years alternating to her house every other weekend to spend time with her. When my mother remarried, I continued to experience an increase in siblings and extended relatives. The contrast of experiencing two different families, an increase of responsibility, and my role in each family was an extremely challenging dynamic to adjust to for many years.

The split family scenario was quite an ongoing change for some time, and it felt like a huge shift of the attention that was once directed solely on me was redirected elsewhere to many others. In no way was anyone doing anything unloving, and it was just a different experience than the life I was living prior as an only child.

I remember before all the changes, I kneeled to pray, asking for siblings because I had wanted someone to play with. I can thankfully say that that prayer was answered! I feel grateful for the unique experience in how I was raised and the contrast in a culture that it gave me. A lot of lessons towards independence began due to the family dynamics. This led to adulthood with frustration, especially how different growing up was for me versus my siblings.

Deep within me, I desired to love and have harmony with everyone, but I always felt out of place, never fully expressing and genuinely felt anyone understood. It pained me to feel such a separation from others because of the unique circumstance. It wasn't easy to shift between families. I felt my internal pressure to show up and please everyone, all while always feeling a bit left out since I couldn't be there for all the family gatherings and had to alternate holidays knowing I was missing out elsewhere.

The constant fluctuation of always having to choose someone vs. another was hard on my spirit. I struggled with communicating with my mother about the difficulties because it was unfair to choose between one family. I felt disempowered and confused on how to handle a situation that didn't seem fair to anyone. I began to focus on school activities and built a strong desire to adventure outside of my hometown to gain freedom and life experience.

After leaving to attend college, I had no idea what was waiting around the corner. One of the hardest lessons was when I moved away and met an older man that completely triggered something I had never felt before. The physical chemistry was so intense that I suddenly found myself in a relationship with a narcissist that had become toxic mentally, emotionally, and eventually physically abusive.

At the time, I didn't realize how dangerous the relationship was, and I kept a lot of it to myself due to the overwhelming confusion of manipulation and control I was in. That was a time of deep pain, yet towards the end of that relationship, the inner growth and connecting to a higher power is what saved me and ultimately changed me to the core. At the time, I had no idea the impact that relationship would have long term. After safely leaving that situation, it inevitably led me to embrace life fully with beautiful experiences once I was free from that attachment.

I spent years afterward on an inward personal self-discovery, self-love journey. I began working on an independent life while struggling along the way. Still, with the mindset of sheer resilience to grow and be authentic to my path, all while remaining in the sense of openness to connect to whomever I'd meet with acceptance and love. I truly love to connect with everyone, whether it's a quick conversation, a smile in passing, or a synchronistic experience that links me to them. How I approach life allows me to remain in alignment, leading me towards directions that connect so organically. I truly believe that's why and how I was able to connect to Radhaa.

One of the beautiful things about connecting online is you can link with people from all over the world, and you don't necessarily have to know them in person. I knew after some time Radhaa's energy was so genuine, wise, and inviting. I saw her as representing how I felt inside and what felt like a sister to me. She's someone who helps me remember who I am, supports, and empowers me.

I felt I was meant to be a Pillar of Light in my heart, and I feel grateful we connected. I love diving deep and connecting to the Creator and seeing the magic in life. Every part of my journey has led me to this point where I was ready to experience a massive shift in my life, and I didn't know how that would look.

When Radhaa and I connected, I knew divine timing was in my heart, and this was the moment! I was ready to elevate and be fully rooted into receiving the Goddess Activations™. I am overwhelmed with gratitude to have been divinely connected to this experience. It was so thrilling that it brought out my inner playful child as she began the session and an overwhelming sense of excitement to connect to the essence of who I am unapologetic.

My soul was screaming, "I am ready!" I felt supported during the session and confident that my journey has led me to the "now" I was about to experience. This process has been about surrendering to the process, deeply trusting myself, and loving myself and others as an extension of the love I have within. It is truly the essence of love, beauty, relationships, abundance, and receptivity.

I knew in my heart the Goddess I felt most connected to was Aphrodite. Once Radhaa connected me to my Goddess, it was Aphrodite that came through! The entire journey was very visual, and I felt Radhaa saw exactly what I was visualizing as she began guiding the process.

I felt Aphrodites essence come through and saw a vision of being in the clouds seeing a beautiful, gentle, and graceful presence that extended a light pink glass heart out to me. Aphrodite welcomed me with a gift, and it gave me such pleasure to receive confirmation that I am a part of the lineage of Venus. It felt so natural to embrace the energy that came forward, yet I was still questioning if I was ever good enough!

I was given a sense of encouragement to embody this essence because Aphrodite knew I struggled with my worthiness. Aphrodite walked side-by-side with me, and I leaned my head on her shoulder, surrendering to this welcome. She gracefully laughed and said, "You're one of us." She was connecting with me like a sister, and I instantly knew what she was saying to me: "You know who you are, so embrace your natural beauty and be rooted in confidence and self-love. You have all the power you need inside of you."

It was a kind, gentle reminder in what felt like a moment of sudden realization that I no longer needed to question my worthiness, but to receive, which at that moment was also very much needed, like subconscious permission to be myself going forward. To my logical mind! I felt supported and embraced the experience while fighting off old feelings of not "feeling worthy" to a deep understanding of just how worthy I've ALWAYS been.

Aphrodite acknowledged the emotional pain I was carrying in my womb from my ancestors and advised a few rituals to help clear the energy from my lineage. It has never been done before, creating a sense of disempowerment and holding old emotional pain no longer needed. The essence of Aphrodite had been trying to connect for years, and in this Activation, I received her Golden light Activation.

As Radhaa continued her channeling Aphrodite, the Goddess expressed to me, "I'm on a divine mission that is guided every step of the way. I am here to usher in Light, Peace, Love, and Harmony and have been commissioned by the Divine to do so." Clearing the old paradigm allows me to step into the new, which is a huge reason I've come here on a soul mission. "This is the end of the old and beginning of the new," she informed me.

As a co-creator, I support others with hope and trust the process by doing what is more aligned with me on a soul level. Aphrodite asked me to release all that does not belong to me, to let go, and to tap into the crystalline rose quartz heart as Radhaa led me on.

The darkness has been consuming the earth. Yet, the crystalline heart light shines out into the world with love, peace, and hope. Radhaa, a conduit of Goddess Aphrodite, placed a golden shield of light around me after she cleansed and cleared me. As I bring forth peace, I stand on the bridge and help those unsure of stepping forward. During the day, I help people come into the world of healing, and at night I help people cross the rainbow bridge. It was confirmed that Radhaa and I have a soul contract to help me remember who I am, which confirms the divine timing of this Activation.

This journey of the Goddess activations™ created a sensation of peace within my essence and an absolute sigh of relief to let go of the prior pain and challenges. It was as though I no longer needed to struggle internally anymore. A sort of internal peace offering to "Be" me, so I can allow all my desires to come forward while just sitting back and "being" myself!

I noticed that I lacked receptivity before the session, which ignited inside of me during this session. It was like meeting with an old friend that reminds you of who you are while graciously lifting your spirits and allowing you to see and feel your value once again. It has energetically helped clear some old patterns within my family lineage and helped bridge my mother's loving connection. It truly has brought a lot of compassion for her to my being. The session was a lighthearted experience that brought so much joy and confirmation to me.

I had been feeling the call of Aphrodite for quite a while and had many personal subtle experiences that connected me to this point in life to the essence of Aphrodite. As a dreamer metaphorically and in my dream state, I had a few dreams that Aphrodite sent me an "energetic alert." Even a year or so before the Activation, this energy connected within me, trying to get my attention.

I had dreamt I was living in a huge house that appeared to be a large mansion with pillars. The home was on the edge of a cliff that led to the ocean. It was a bright clear day with no clouds in sight. The property's surroundings felt like I lived in a peaceful, happy environment with a very well-maintained landscape. Pristine space surrounding me included a pool in the backyard area where I was lounging around. I suddenly saw myself swinging on one of those tall swings. I began to swing partially over the backyard property then over the cliff above the ocean. I could feel the cool breeze as I was swinging peacefully back and forth while feeling incredibly blissful. As I leaned back, I could see my long, tan, skinny legs pointing to the sky and a glimpse of the sheer dress I was wearing flowing through the air as I swung over the ocean below and back to land. I was alone, spending quality time with myself while observing my surroundings. This was a dream that felt like one of the most amazing dreams I've ever had! I typically dream of many people or dream of experiencing some other community activity that's generally not about me. This one was unique, and I felt the Goddess was coming through in my dream!

A year or so later, another synchronistic dream occurred. Details I cannot remember, but I do remember the most important part. It was a spiritual dream where I was fighting something/someone and felt an inner power of authority as a command saying, "I am the bringer of light!" I felt like I was battling while standing up for truth, a strong feeling of the embodiment of my inner power with the command to whomever I was speaking to. This dream always left me feeling the inner power to claim my sovereignty. An intense command of embodiment carried from my dream state into my physical reality immediately upon awakening.

At the time of the dream, I had no idea how this was all connected. After learning about Aphrodite, I learned that Venus could observe the naked eye at dawn and dusk. Venus has always been the light-bringer as it always precedes the early morning sun, and it is the brightest planet in the Solar System. The ancient Greeks had named the bright star Aphrodite in honor of their most beautiful Goddess. Goddess Aphrodite's name stems from a word meaning: Shining, Wonder, and Bright.

Following the Activation and some integration of the codes, I realized the essence of Aphrodite had been communicating to me in my sleep leading up to the Activation.

The essence is already inside me, but I received small golden threads leading up to help wake me up to the deeper levels of my consciousness and the importance of this Activation. It is how some wake up to higher states of reality over a duration of time. Synchronicity is here and there for you to process and discern along your journey. I see synchronicities as small keys to the wake-up call and growth in our conscious evolution.

Looking back on past relationships, I realize it's all about stepping into my power, trusting my intuition and independence while maintaining a healthy relationship with myself as I build relationships with others. The shadow aspect I had been working through to clear, an obsessive passion that completely took over me negatively, greatly affected my self-esteem. There are levels to this, and when I connected to Radhaa, I was on the edge of a revisited lesson testing me to be sure I was ready to level up. Letting go and leaning into receptivity hadn't always been easy for me, but due to divine timing, the Goddess Activations™ modality helped guide me through with the help of Aphrodite.

Following the session, I found I had made a forward movement. Still, I felt something was holding me energetically to a specific individual in my heart, which kept me in old patterns of self-sacrifice, lack of worthiness, and doubting my intuition due to conflicting inner feelings vs. what was happening in the physical world.

As Radhaa began the next session, I told her I was still dealing with this deep yearning of an attachment to a specific person in my life, and I must clear this. After discussing what was coming up for me, we both knew it was time to do an energetic divorce to release the old energies of a past timeline. I was still carrying the contract and loyalty of that past life marriage. The process was overwhelming at first because I could feel the connection in my body and struggled with letting go with resistance in my heart. Still, I also knew it was time to surrender and trusted I was following through on my lesson learned from this lifetime. As she started walking me through the process, I began to cry.

Radhaa asked what was coming up for me, and I said I shouldn't be doing this. I feel a strong sense of "loyalty." "The energy had been carried over into this lifetime, a loyal commitment to that individual," says Radhaa. Radhaa had seen our life together, and it was a very happy, fulfilling life of equally shared love. She walked me through a process, and it was very touching to know, my soul chose to evolve past that timeline, and he supported it by telling me, "Go ahead, honey, I'll catch up. I love you." It was brought to the Creator to be released, and we began clearing old cords. I instantly stopped crying and felt a huge shift of that energy release from my body. I felt lighter and had more space in my body. I could breathe down into my chest the moment I felt the shift. The release of the old energetic cords that are not mine to carry in this lifetime dissolved the strong feelings of commitment which released what felt like attachment.

It was a beautiful process. To assist with the shift, Radhaa brought in Quan Yin. She stepped forward to help with Aphrodite. I am so grateful for the assistance of this nurturing and comforting Goddess during a time of grief and sorrow of letting go.

My soul remembered our life together and recognized his eyes when we first met, and I always felt like I had a strong connection, as though I was in a relationship with him in my heart. Since the shift, I have worked on my boundaries and letting go to bring forward the essence of Aphrodite into the new version of me as Danielle in this lifetime. It takes great inner strength and the willingness to do the work of healing myself and my lineage to ascend in consciousness. Thankfully, Radhaa knows how to hold sacred space and truly get to the root of the situation at hand.

A few weeks after working to anchor in the Pillar of Light and bring forward a brighter essence of Aphrodite, I started to get exhausted physically. I had felt my energy had been unusually tiresome. When I spoke to Radhaa about it, she scanned my energy field and instantly knew what was happening. She saw an ancient entity attached to me that was taking my life force energy. It was putting me into a state of hypnotic sedation, causing me to need sleep. I felt exhausted and had no motivation of any sort.

Radhaa helped remove and send this entity back to the Creator with the help of Sekhmet, Durga, and Akhilandishwari. Aphrodite stepped in to help provide healing with her beautiful light pink energy. This season helped me solidify how important this work is and how trusting yourself is very important during the process. I knew something was off but wasn't sure what had been happening. This energy can be very detrimental to one's health and bring dis-ease into life. It is not something to fear but to become conscious of the energies that affect our energetic field and subconscious.

Aphrodite came in to share how important Rose Quartz was for me with healing. Rose Quartz has great healing properties for the mind, body, and spirit. It belongs to the "Great Mother" stones and links your heart to the earth and the whole cosmos. Its soft color works with your broken heart, and the essence covers your body with vibrations that heal ailments of the heart and circulatory system. It's what I needed after the grief of an old love and an unexpected entity that had been plaguing my family for a very long time. It is confirmation that I must continue to trust myself and listen to the whispers and synchronicities in my life. It also brought awareness in spiritual hygiene and a Protection Prayer I now say daily, which Radhaa also provided me.

Following the sessions, I have become more trusting of my intuition. I have been increasingly in alignment, and it brings so much pleasure and love to the moment I'm currently in. My creative inspiration has increased, and my sense of knowing my value and making choices that reflect that have become a priority to honor my integrity with myself and others. I see so much potential for growth with the support of Aphrodite as I become a better version of my future self going forward daily. I feel so much love and empathy for all and how much we as a collective go through that deserves love.

Aphrodite Goddess Activations™ experience has helped me identify my values and where I need to make changes to create the balance of masculine and feminine for humanity within myself. I have more of a realization that our dream state creates our dreams in the physical world. Aphrodite reminds me of my inner power to anchor peace, love, embody worthiness, and provide hope for the emerging of the Heaven we're anchoring to Earth as Pillars of Light. My experience with Goddess Activations™ led me back home to trust myself and always follow the golden threads of my heart.

∼

Saying:

"Individually and collectively, we are shifting from a position of fear into surrender and trust of the intuitive. The power of the feminine energy is on the rise in our world."

~ Shakti Gawain

DANIELLE SCHRECK

~ CONTRIBUTING WRITER ~

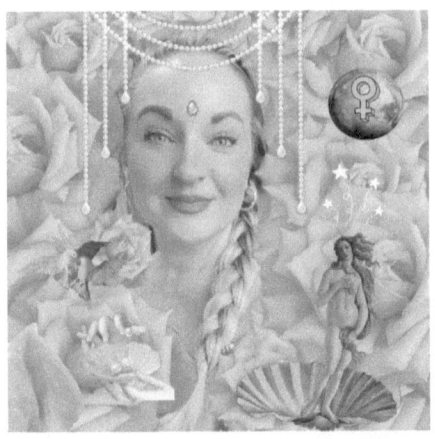

Danielle Schreck is Certified in Spinning Goddess Pendulum Healing Course at Goddess Code Academy. She's an Empath that loves connecting with people. She specializes in podcasts and interviews for holistic healers. Her background is in the corporate world. Her inner passion is exploring spirituality, personal development, and seeking to connect more with others. She focuses on following her heart to bridgework her personal life to serve the Creator. She enjoys expanding-deep conversations, painting, and enjoying peaceful time in nature. Find Danielles Aphrodite Heart Vibes Store here: https://etsy.me/3DGIlUS

Saying:

"The rise of the Divine Feminine does not have to be at the expense of the Sacred Masculine. It is about the complete respect of the differences that the Sacred Masculine and Divine Feminine bring to a physical and spiritual union."

~ Reena Kumarasingham

CHAPTER 5

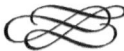

LAKSHMI GODDESS ACTIVATIONS™

Maya Verzonilla, AKA Maya The Shaman

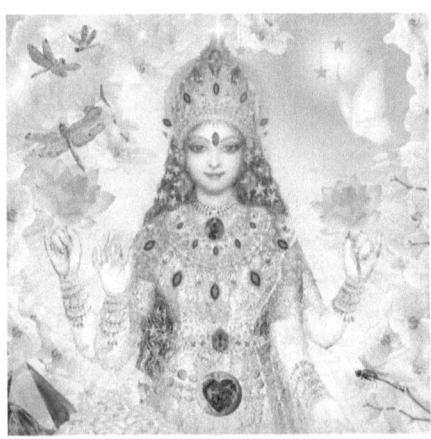

"There is a wonderful world created by a devotee with her Goddess. Spiritually and traditionally in the East, these two celebrates each other's bonding through unconditional devotion provided by a devotee to her Goddess (or God.) In return, the Goddess unconditionally provide gifts back to her devotee."
~ *Maya Verzonilla*

Devotee and The Goddess

I always have this attraction and love for the Goddesses. There are several Goddesses that I have been drawn to, one of them is Goddess Lakshmi. Connecting with my Goddess of choice through the guidance of Radhaa as a conduit and Goddess Activator is a precious experience I look forward to share.

Being a Shaman and a healer myself, I am so used to being the giver of sessions. It was refreshing to relax and receive cosmic downloads of abundance from this sacred session.

Radhaa asked me to be in a comfortable position. She instructed me to sit or lie down. I have chosen to lie down as this is always the best and soothing way to allow a powerful healing transformation to take place. As I got ready for the first three breaths which Radhaa had asked me to begin with, my body easily got settled, waiting to meet my Goddess.

Sacred Space - Lakshmi Goddess Activations™

Radhaa went into the sacred space of the Source of All that Is. I felt a warm and glowing cocoon of love where my Spiritual Guides were standing by my side and stayed throughout this entire session with me. I felt a feeling of surrendering myself to this experience. I know intuitively that this is one of those special moments I would have another mystical encounter. So I happily allowed and looked forward to Goddess Lakshmi's presence in this Pillars of Light, Goddess Activations™.

Radhaa is a Master of her Goddess Activations™. Please know that in this type of work, if the healer or the conduit is not knowing how to connect to the supreme consciousness, the sentient energy of the Divine, there can potentially be sabotaged by the dark forces (entities of all kinds). I have witnessed it. Having a spiritual guide who knows exactly how to connect with a true Goddess will make anyone feel safe. As I deeply relaxed within the space held by Radhaa, I breathed deeply.

Radhaa's voice was soothing and I went deeper into a meditative state, hearing Radhaa speak. I entered a sort of lucid state of consciousness. Her voice was soft, rhythmic, and Angelic. Soon Radhaa has invited Goddess Lakshmi to come to our session. I saw Goddess Lakshmi before me. Lakshmi came with her open arms and loving presence. She is fully adorned with her gold jewels, gold coins pouring from her energetic field, and the golden light is all around her. I felt as if her sweet and loving presence communed with me.

<u>Goddess Lakshmi
& Golden Lemurian DNA Activation</u>

In my 3rd eye, I see Radhaa side by side with Goddess Lakshmi. This feeling was so uplifting that I felt the sensation of floating on clouds. I felt very, very light. There were moments I went in and out of this present timeline and space, and time had seemed to stop.

Lakshmi was standing right in front of me as she poured her golden light into me. Lakshmi said she was activating and upgrading my Golden Lemurian DNA. The Golden Lemurian DNA was downloaded to me by the Universe sometime ago, and I used it in my sessions with my clients. This time, I am ready to receive the next upgrade through the Goddess of grace, abundance, and wealth, by Radhaa's method of Goddess Activations™.

The activation continued. Radhaa lovingly held this sacred session for me with Goddess Lakshmi while safely allowing this magic to occur.

As I witnessed this sacred transference, Goddess Lakshmi stretched out her hands once more towards me. Held in her hands were sparks of golden dust like shimmering lights, the powerful advanced Lemurian Code upgrades that she pulled out of the ethers, unfolding the Golden DNA strands in front of me. Then, she said that this is for me, towards the sacred work that I have been doing. A gift of offering by a Goddess which left me stunned and delight.

Goddess Lakshmi told me that these DNA strands would be my upgrade. I felt so honored and so grateful to experience this magical resonance with Goddess Lakshmi. As we heal and activate, we can hold more and more light. And this Goddess Activations™ by Radhaa is truly one of those precious gifts from the Divine.

Radhaa's voice came in and out continuously as I drifted into another realm. Then Goddess Lakshmi started to tell me about the many projects I am to create. As Radhaa spoke, I sometimes heard her voice and other times fading away. I felt like my space had expanded. At this moment, I was floating into a vast space of cosmic consciousness and a trance-like state of being, which I often go into. It accompanied me in a state of letting it be.

Goddess Lakshmi continued to downpour her unconditional love and blessings. This time, explaining further that we as humanity are going through this passage, from dark to light. The Goddess continued to say, "the work you do as a Lemurian Code Healer is very important, intense, and at times can be heavy on you, transmuting darkness into light." I agree, for I knew it. The Goddess knew the truth of my work as a Shaman. I have encountered many heavy loads that I have held for my family and clients to assist them in their journey of upgrading their consciousness and DNA. Being a Lemurian Code healer and the holder of the "Infinite Cosmic Records," Goddess Lakshmi knew that so many people needed my assistance at this time.

This advanced golden DNA upgrade that Goddess Lakshmi gifted me with is truly aligned with my work as a Shaman Healer. Goddess Lakshmi guided me on a step-by-step divine plan of what will be on my plate and how exactly to manifest this work with her grace.

I was surprised how much the Goddess wanted me to be more patient in doing this work, and so the Goddess handed me a long list of to-do items, but it made perfect sense. Goddess Lakshmi mentioned that for the moment, I am working on the most intense timeline, but soon it would lead to a whole lot more new realm filled with lightness and joy, she added.

Soon after, the gold coins come down pouring like waterfalls from her hands. The Goddess said that the new creative work I would do would be blissful, and energy would flow through the projects I am working on.

Orbs, Flying Dolphins & Unicorns

Radhaa's conduit work with Goddess Lakshmi continued beautifully and magically. Radhaa was with me, seeing everything the entire time, holding sacred space. She spoke of it while I saw it manifest. Magenta orbs of light gently floated, levitating around me, in a very peaceful ambiance. Lakshmi told me that these were the original mystical orbs from Lemuria. They were the guardians of this sacred land at the beginning of time, and they still exist. Lakshmi placed one of the orbs in my heart chakra. I felt a wave of remembrance and gratitude. Visions came; the once upon a time landscape of the ancient past, the time during the era of paradise in Lemuria, dolphins, whales, dragons, and magical creatures. Then, a vision of the shimmering light and colorful landscape appeared. A true haven and sanctuary on Earth that once carried a higher octave and frequency created by the original land keepers of Mu, showed up. A place of such mystical beings who came from the heart of the Universe and landed on Mother Earth, who equally matched the same high octave during the time of Mu appeared in front of me. I felt its magic, and it felt like everything was lit up with luminescent light.

This beautiful purple orb continued to hover around my space and within me. Then I had visions about myself in Lemuria in a total state of abundance. Everything was lit up again with bright, colorful light. Gold was abundant and was easy to access. The original abundance of enchanted Mother Earth, pristine paradise was in Mu. Lemuria and Mu were the same names pointing to the lost continent of the Pacific, Maharlika (the Philippines). It was like watching a virtual screen, and it felt so real. Lakshmi was connecting me back to a part of myself that is eternally abundant. She said that later on I would be sharing these magical teachings with others.

I felt like her presence was filling up my half-filled cup because I was exhausted from all the mundane activities before this session arrived, and the Goddess was asking me to let the tiredness go and simply be in the state of receiving.

Soon, Goddess Lakshmi started to show me the flying dolphins. Yes, they had magnificent, iridescent, and translucent wings! Then Unicorns came after. They came into my space and started to communicate with me. At that moment, I was again in and out of a lucid state, a dream-like reality.

When the Unicorns started communicating with me, they repeated their message three times! Over and over again, they would say something like this," Remember Who You are! Remember Who You are! Remember Who You are!" It made me laugh out loud! They made so much sense, but they were hilarious and full of this bubbly, light energy that tickled my heart.

Goddess Lakshmi continued to share with me that these Unicorns were once part of Lemuria. And that they exist. As the world continues to degenerate in consciousness, they have moved into the higher realms, as most magical and mystical beings have done to preserve themselves. Goddess Lakshmi instructed me "to never forget them, that they are a part of Lemuria's family. She added that "I am a keeper of Unicorn energy and essence, and this would be a part of my sacred work." I chuckled. Because, in some ways, I do love unicorns, but had forgotten them for some time now. Yet, when my kids were little, I got Unicorn stuffed toys for them, and it was one of the favorite toys my daughter enjoyed.

So many moon years have passed, and the Unicorn energy is coming back into my life again through Goddess Lakshmi's grace. It feels childlike and a very sweet reminder of fond memories. It made me feel light in contrast to the intense work I do at times. As a Shaman, I dealt with suicidal clients, addicts, life and death situations, clients who have had dark magic sent to them, so many people with heavy baggage and much intensity where issues are not near light. Some clients have told me that I am their very last hope. At times, it's a lot of pressure because I hold the container of my work very seriously. I've never regretted serving my clients in a sacred space with a great deal of love and compassion because this is an inner-calling type of work I do. But working with their heavy karma can be taxing on my body. And do you know that authentic indigenous Shamans like myself hold these weights in our bodies to clear? Yes, authentic indigenous Shamans swallow poisons. They absorb toxins and process them for others! It is hard to still believe such an act in our modern age, but the sacrifice made by authentic Shamans are different from the dark workers. The Light-worker Shamans sacrifice themselves, while the Minions of the Dark sacrifice others, through human trafficking, etc. and covered humanity with the 'blanket of darkness.'

Shamanic Transmutation

It is to be known that indigenous Shamans transmute so much into their vessels to assist others in releasing darkness, so light can come through them. I am like a sponge, and I absorb the energy of all types from those I come in contact with. Yes, many authentic Shamans sacrifice their lives in this work of helping others move through their darkness to get back into the light. I love my work. I love my clients. But I admit that there are times it's like lifting heavy weights, and with so many people counting on me to assist them on their journey, it can be exhausting, yet, I am honored and happy to be of service. In this year 2022 and beyond, I affirm to lighten my load and follow Lakshmi's advice, lighten up!

With Goddess Lakshmi by my side, I am reminded of the lightness of being, which is the original template and lightness of our Spirit. I am reminded to be a joyful Shaman.

Goddess Lakshmi showed me what is installed in my future. Even while doing this intense work as a Shaman, I can be playful, she said, lightness of heart is my natural state of being. Such reminder is so priceless. For me, I value Goddess Lakshmi's gifts as sacred gems from the Universe. She ask me to shine bright—be in joy! It is the best gift ever —a soulful gift of reminder!

A Spa for the Soul

To receive this Goddess Activations™ from Radhaa is like going into a high-end Spa for the Soul. I felt like I was massaged, pampered, and rejuvenated on the deepest levels. Goddess Activations™ has lit up my Spirit into a deeper and more pleasant remembering. Another rich layer of this experience with Goddess Activations™, enhancing my devotion to Goddess Lakshmi. She appeared with her powerful gifts, the Lemurian Golden DNA advanced activation installed in me, the Lemurian magical ancient spirit animals, and the guidance to shine in joy! And isn't that what we could use more of. I celebrate this sacred encounter, and what a lovely realm!

"Embracing our divine feminine in Indigenous world-views also means honoring time as infinite and cyclical, rather than linear. Mother Earth teaches us to honor rhythms, seasons, rather than always having to be "on", always producing. This honoring of cyclical time allows us to also be more compassionate with self, and with others, as we no longer feel pressure to have to perform on a clock. The absence of external pressure allows you to move with the flow of life, honor what comes, and have compassion as we are able to be more present with what shows up." ~ Dr. Rocio Rosales Meza

I felt fully supported by this amazing Golden Goddess. Lakshmi is truly a Master. I stand as a pillar of light for Lakshmi Goddess Activations™. As her devotee, she provided her unconditional boon! I am especially grateful to Radhaa, the conduit of this majestic, all-inspiring modality! It is a must to experience Goddess Activations™. Radhaa is truly a Goddess Activator! Thank you, Radhaa. And thank you, Goddess Lakshmi. I'm forever grateful!

∾

MAYA VERZONILLA

~ CONTRIBUTING WRITER ~

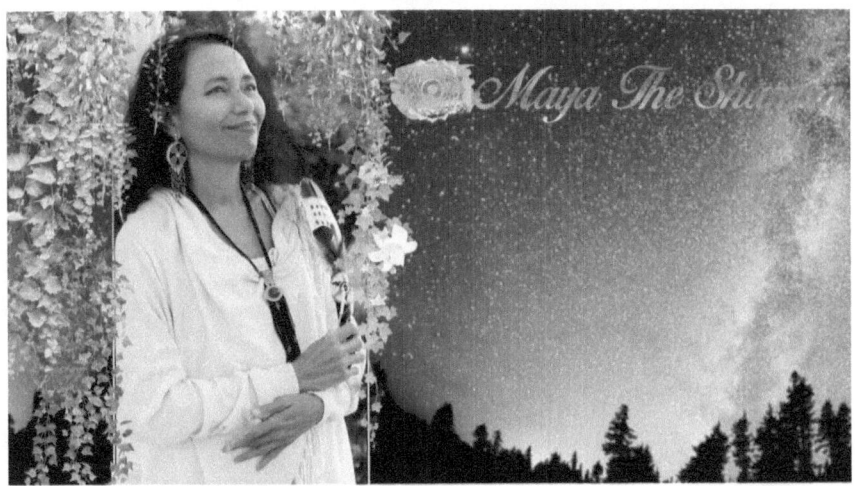

Maya Verzonilla, AKA *Maya The Shaman,* is an indigenous Shaman-Healer from Maharlika (the Philippines) living at the Appalachian mountains of the Carolinas.

She is a Creative Writing Coach, and Co-Author of the Best-Selling "*Awakening Starseeds*" book series.

Maya's upcoming collaborative books 2022 are: "Energy Healing & Soul Medicine" (Spring), "Awakening Starseeds: Dreaming into the Future Vol. 3" (Summer), and a stand alone book, "Infinite Cosmic Records: Sacred Doorways to Healing & Remembering" (Summer), a rich-filled stories of Maya and her clients on Shamanic healing guided by Maya during her clients sessions in entering their Cosmic Records with her. Maya's Memoir, "Descendants of Lemuria," will be released on 2023,

Maya also appeared in several documentary films: "The Cure," Produced by actress, Sharon Stone and French Director Manuel Itier. Another docu-film she was asked to take part was "Guns Bombs & War: A Love Story," were cries on Earth wars — crime against humanity. Maya's involvement in these films is to assist humanity to heal and move forward into our Golden Age, where Peace, Health, and Freedom are our Sovereign Rights.

Lemurian Code Healing and *Infinite Cosmic Records,* are original healing modalities by Maya The Shaman. To learn more about Certification Programs, please contact Maya at: lemuriancodehealing@gmail.com or www.LemurianShaman.com

CHAPTER 6

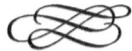

SARASWATI GODDESS ACTIVATIONS™

Anna Lieberman

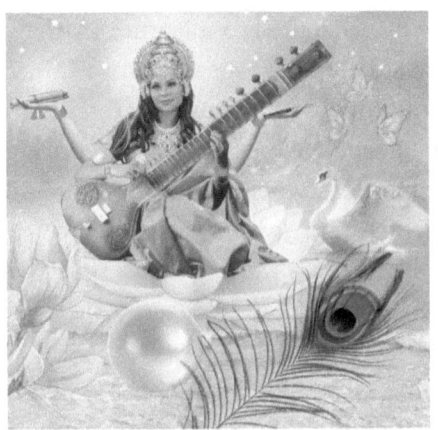

Anchoring Saraswati

"Is that a Peacock?!" I yelled out loud to no one, slamming on my brakes, coming to a complete halt on a busy two-lane street in Pasadena, Ca. The Peacock sauntered on like a twenty-something-year-old who knows how hot they are, literally and happily stopping traffic. My jaw dropped as I fumbled to open the camera while muttering, "there's fucking..Peacocks..?! just like..in the street now?"

Not long after the Peacock crossed the road, I felt guided to work with Radhaa.

"I sense Saraswati....anchor Her," was Radhaas's response, paraphrased. And I hadn't told her about the Peacock yet, but I didn't need to. Radhaa has a vision, and she can see me, cloak or no cloak. Saraswati is often depicted alongside a peacock or swan.

But let's back up a little.

A Brief Introduction

Saraswati is inflow, the Goddess of true knowledge and wisdom, speech, sound, mantra, and music, to return dignity to and empower the individual through full authentic expression. Her presence enlivens and empowers us through creation.

Suppose you've ever listened to a lecture by the late great Terrence Mckenna, the psychedelic Shakespeare himself. In that case, you can feel Her embrace of him as he weaves new realities into being through improvisational language. She is easily felt through Lauryn Hill in "The Mystery of Iniquity, "where true wisdom finds a way into the world through divinely creative expression. She is most present in those moments witnessing an artist whose gift is out of this world, jaw-dropping; how'd they do that? Best believe they're communing with Saraswati.

I've been working with, beseeching, and embodying Saraswati for as long as I can remember. My relationship with Her is perhaps the most fulfilling and rewarding connection to the divine I have experienced to date. Entering a flow state in the presence of Saraswati is as magical as a unicorn on acid. It's butterfly sex. It's a guitar solo that can make you orgasm. The spirit of Saraswati reminds me of magic mushrooms quite a bit. It's surpassing the frontal lobes and landing in a pure being. There's no doubt in it, no doublethink, no critical psychoanalysis. It's alive with theatrical passion, sometimes comical, other times enraged, never judging the moment, too busy being in it. Our emotional bodies and imaginations, under the tutelage of Saraswati, alchemize into cosmically aligned purpose. She's an absolute riot and hugely underrated in modern culture, which tends to worship her sister Lakshmi. Do you want to know a secret, though? Saraswati is back, baby, and she's stepping into the light now — a moment the whole Earth can celebrate together.

Mantra

Heaviness of life surrender unto mantra grace AUM NAMAH SHIVAYA

Weave breathe in retention
Chant
AUM
NAMAH
SIVAYA
Supreme Mantra Deeksha
Liberated in Consciousness the Yogi Be!
Nandhiji (author of Mastery of Consciousness) (Albums: Cave of the Siddhars)

Saraswati is the Goddess of mantra, music, and sound vibrations—their invisible albeit undeniable effect on the space around and within us. Sound vibrations have immense, inherent power to ripple in space, changing it— and they don't stop at our bodies, and they go right through us, touching every cell. We can feel it as these vibrations activate motion in the body, spark emotion, conjure release, make us weep, or put us to sleep, amongst other things.

Meeting mantra as a westerner for the first time was an enlightening experience, and so naturally, it was also enigmatic and brain-stretching. It was like being given a telephone directory to the cosmos and then sent on my way with a smile and a wink, haha! A dear friend invited me to participate in a Puja with Naandhii. I didn't know what a

Puja was, or what mantra was, or anything about Indian culture, spiritual practices, mythology. I was going in blind, and I had been invited to do so. After an evening of fumbling through foreign syllables like my mouth had too much food in it, dancing in circles beneath the Sages gone before, placing single petals of a flower on altars with acute intention and being called to the attention of inter-dimensional oneness, the mantra was on my radar. This was the initiation of my Voice, and I didn't even know it! It takes time to see.

>   Reeng Ung Ong Ganapatye Namah
>   And
>   Govinda Go
>   And
>   Aum ari Aum
>   And
>   Aum Namah Sivaya...
>   ....rang in my ears like a phantom echo.

I could hardly bring myself to utter the words out loud. I felt silly. I felt stupid. I felt like a spirit would pop out of the wall and yell, "CULTURAL APPROPRIATOR! YOU FUCKING WHITE LADY CLICHÉ!" I did it anyway, trusting the purity of my heart was visible in the divine realms. I started using the beads Naandhi gave me that night. I wrote out the name he gave me as he signed and dedicated a copy of his book to me: "Sivayani Devi, feb 28 2019 Ariven."

In the time, it was the mantras who came knocking at my door while I'd practice on my instrument (a Baritone Ukulele) as a mother knocked on the door of her sad teenage daughter. With a little rub on the back and some encouragement from Saraswati, I opened my mouth. Finally, the mantra intersected this desire. I've always had to let my Voice run without the need for lyrics, without talking words as per yooshj. When chanting, the mouth is given its task but doesn't require the same kind of attention from the mind, allowing it to open like a lotus. Whoa.

I'd pick two or three chords and a mantra with resonance at the moment- intuitively- and I'd sing them on repeat, like a chorus on loop x108. The purpose of a practice like this is not to top the charts or be a Pop Star, though no judgment upon that path. Go Billie, Free Britney. Something more interesting and mysterious to me was going on than fame and notoriety, something more enticing than storming the music scene. The potential to enter an expanded, meditative headspace, for example. A doorway into flow state into other realms and dimensions! Alchemy, transmutation, energy work, it's all there awaiting discovery. Some sessions ended in weeping; healings were taking place spontaneously, downloads were happening, my understanding began to grow and grow and grow. What remains inside the mystery today, I couldn't tell you.

"Holllyyyy SHIT!" said I, after any given session of chanting.

Saraswati takes me by the hand and says with amusement, lighting her eyes, "Come on I'll show you around your Voice. I'll show you how music is energy." I began to make sounds I'd never made before as I entered new levels of awareness about the vibrations my vocal cords were making in my body and the physiology surrounding it—what it feels like in my jaw, my throat, my chest, my nose, my crown, my mind, heart, and spirit, too; what the breath is doing, the feeling of support in the diaphragm, all these things functioning together without a single concentrated thought. How sublime. In many ways, not unlike a vocal coach or learning the basics of singing, however, with the greeting of self in presence set as priority overmastering a skill, well, a mysterious difference in the experience emerges. There's a new liberation in it. There's no need or pressure to sound good. The purpose of the practice will live and thrive no matter what you sound like. Try it sometime. Vocalize with the reckless abandon of the outcome and instead revel in the experience of creating vibration within your beautiful body, gliding on each breath.

Soon after I began practicing came the sensation of becoming a channel that I can describe as being sung, the same way I am danced as Dakini. A voice will with character presents itself out of nowhere through its vowels, the shape of the mouth, and the amount and placement of the breath. Without thought, a new sound comes in like a jazz solo, and I applaud them when they go, shake my head up and down, smiling... "Cool, nice. Haha, what was that?" It's often surprising, and you can feel it when you've fallen out of it. The ability to enter and sustain this space grows in the ease with practice.

It was a peculiar and elusive discovery. How, "ok, I sang it, right? but...is that one my Voice? Is that..me.. or?" And if so, then are all of them my Voice? I could cut 20 albums with each persona if I wanted to, so what shall I do with this? Tell me each of you your heart's desire. I adapted further and began using English at times. I listen with huge grins to my peers around the globe on this same frequency who are doing the same thing I am in their way, like the stunning "Mantras in Love" by the Goddess Pack "Beautiful Chorus" who chant:

> Be here now
> And
> Within Me is Boundless Love
> And
> Thank You...

...all of which are sung in sweet, simple harmony. You can feel their collective flow space. It's so beautiful and powerful! A gift to the ears it enters.

Often I'll make a mantra up on the spot, tailored to my current state. Like:

> Dear one I am here for you
> I am grateful for my life.
> Or
> I am a morning person.
> Or
> I feel comfortable in crowded places
> I am not addicted to coffee
> I am unphased when he doesn't text me back. That's fine. It's fine.
> I jest. AND YET!

Though I enjoy adapting and weaving this ancient, sacred Indian modality with the language I was born into, I most often enter a chant with my head bowed in reverence, inviting Her presence to come forth as She please, be it intentionally sanctimonious, profane, solemn, salacious, she'll let me know, and then we'll go. And we'll mean it.

This practice most influenced and inspired, beckoned, motivated, and supported the creation of my music. I created Baby Elephants Flow Journal to usher the experiences into the physical and offer my expressions lasting existence here. Soon I had boatloads of music coming through me, transforming me in the process, guiding and aiding me on my healing journey as the mystery deepens ever on.

> "...fulfilled desires to be the fire of wholeness,
> seeking even greater wholeness is in the mantra.."
> Naandhiji

Enter Radhaa Stage Left

Before I tell you about Radhaa, I must fill you in on Zen, her brother. I've now had the joy of collaborating alongside both members of this Power Sibling Situation and find it noteworthy that I have an experience inclusive of a masculine expression mirroring Radhaa's feminine. Also worth mentioning is the context within which I met Zen, a story of the past wherein the very pattern I'm seeking to resolve for good with Radhaa at present was at work then. The link is clear.

This theme, introduced through trauma, which I've sought to overcome for many years, was in full force, and it's to do with my Voice. It was a time of darkness back then with Zen, which is not a bad time. There's a difference. The darkness, the unconscious, it's merely the not knowing exactly what is going on. So you inquire about it. Maybe you panic about it, run away from it screaming at first, but that's not sustainable. It's like walking into an empty football stadium in pitch black, with a triple aaa battery-powered plastic flashlight and trying to find your purse. And you can't leave without your keys, so there's no way around this unless you abandon your vehicle, and your vehicle represents your soul, so, hi, I'm a special ops dark worker with a specialization in light. El gusto es mio, ya dig?

I didn't know at the time, but I can tell you that I realized my inability to speak up for myself with the grace of hindsight and hindsight of grace. I had been robbed of my Voice, and I had amnesia about it. Furthermore, I tended to find myself buddying up with energies that would happily control, dominate and silence me. It was uncomfortable and perplexing, to say the least because I'd been a leader for as long as I could remember, so cognitive dissonance to the maximum with strong indications of unprocessed trauma is my present self's understanding of my precious past self.

In this early, ten years ago, when most everything was tumultuous and difficult, Zen lives in my memory as a trustworthy space of safety. He successfully mediated the shadow masculine and feminine at play and somehow managed to avert impending sabotage at every step. I regard him highly as an awakened being and a brilliant artist, and it is through my relationship with him, I became aware of Radhaa, his sister.

We started to follow each other, Radhaa and I, on social media and have consistently supported one another with likes and comments for I don't know how many years, but you can feel the difference in energy coming from true mutual support, friendship and respect as opposed to those energies animated by ulterior motives. Radhaa's always been the former, sharing herself, offering her gifts, sans solicitation or manipulation; so sovereign and consistent. I've enjoyed witnessing her embodiments of Goddess Archetypes through her gorgeous face and creativity. I mean God, her face, have you seen it? It's out of this world. The images she creates, herself a living artwork, whisper to parts of me I've tucked safely away, inviting me out of the cave, ensuring me of my safety, all without pressure. There's a sense of teamwork in the air, quite organically. I've been nurtured by her stories, intel, and prayers she shares, as well as her unflinching courage to be boldly herself and stand her ground. These observations are not fluffy flattery but rather an insight into how discerningly I will scan before letting someone within miles of my shit, man. I take a good close look. Who wouldn't, once you know what's up. Ah, the old guard sacred grounds where understanding and an alignment of hearts were undoubtedly necessary and present. This is Radhaas's role to play in my life and the lives of many others—the hand that comes to hold yours and cross the bridge with you, whichever one is for you. How epic. Hey you, you sexy ass wayshower, hey you graceful amalgamation of Her, you fellow STAAAARSEEEED! Thank you. Beep beep, incoming message from @annaliebsy to @Radhaanilia. "Hey, soooo... I'm ready."

My Session With Radhaa

"We don't heal by talking about the past.
We heal by talking about what's alive in us right now. The past stimulated that."
~*Marshall Rosenberg*

For a moment, let's suspend all disbelief together as I show you a moment or two of this work. All that which begs of us to stay in reality we've known for many years since we left childhood behind and became increasingly serious about what is real and what is not, as if we can know for certain, let's leave that by the spectacles and today's paper over there at the breakfast nook. Take two steps to your left, hop up and down three times, say "Aum namah Sivaya." Now look around and see a whole new world. There's more to existence than we can comprehend through the lens of our five senses. Let's decree the presence of multi-sensory beings with expanding abilities to communicate with the cosmos. Radhaa and I being two of such.

We began our session with a brief anecdote from childhood that clues us in to the foundational patterns we're here to change, patterns that link to timelines we're here to clear. We don't stay there, however, with the story, I mean, we don't pull it apart into a thousand thoughts or analyses. Instead, Radhaa begins to create a landscape in the fifth dimension. She's not alone either. Divine presence joins her and me, the symphony of the universe she calls them. It feels like a room full of healers surrounding me. They're pure energy, alive and conscious, taking on form at will.

"Quan Yin is at your back," she says.

I see her take form. I can feel the energy moving into my heart from her palm. In my body, it feels like warmth, and in my mind, it's a voice of understanding. A witness who sees all the grief I haven't spoken, all I'm holding. It feels good, and I lean into it, my head bows, my eyes well, and I feel gratitude. It all happens telepathically in an instant.

We continued to multiple areas of interest, landing in a past life regression with my childhood anecdote. The story haunting me in this life is your basic haters going to hate situations. It's happened so many times this go around, and I'd like it to stop. I adapted by becoming invisible, living quietly and small, using my cloak to stay safe. Which, hey, is not always a bad option. It's kept me alive a time or two. But what if I could end this cycle right now? There's got to be a better way. I'm tired of hiding. So we went back. Way back. Imagine traveling through a black void in your mind's eye until images begin to take shape without any effort. This is how I see such things.

Shackles.
A prison cell
Dark, dank, cold
That's where I was at night
In the morning, I was put in the center of town for humiliation
There's a crowd yelling at me, jeering, spitting

"Why? This doesn't make any sense, this is absurd," were my thoughts, then.

I was in shock and disbelief. I couldn't speak. And then, in the crowd, I saw a familiar face. A face I know today. With every word against me, she grows in favor of this crowd. It's wrong. She hates me. She's vile, laughing, so happy to see me like this. She has everything except the one thing she can't have, my essence. And this drives her mad. So here I am, chained in disgrace. Separated from my family, my children. No, my daughter. I have a daughter. Oh God, help.

I didn't see my death, but I'm sure you could imagine as well as I can.

"Ok, so we're going to do an energetic divorce now." says Radhaa.

Wow. I'm so glad she's here. Relief swept over me like a scene in a movie where a high-powered defense attorney shows up unexpectedly.

Stepping away from the scene of humiliation, I'm now standing in the black void with Radhaa and Athena.

"I'm scanning for the chords. I see it at your sternum, do you see anything else?"

"That's it, that's exactly where it is, the sternum."

"You've been working on this"

"Yes"

"There's been some karmic weaving, some soul stalking."

"Yes!"

She was correctly, intuitively describing the experience with the grace of vision and understanding.

"I'd like for you to say her name and command her into this space."

Have you ever commanded the soul of a person who hurt you to join you in a black void? I hadn't. It feels good. With my chin up, calm, safe, divine support at my back, there I am, ready to straighten this out.

Radhaa then led me in ritual and visualizations. I watched as the chord dissolved off my sternum. I watched as Athena sliced and dissolved this story into particle and wave. (Damn, Athena is badass!) I watched as fragments from each of our beings were pulled into a black fire, zero point, neither good nor bad, to be reset, what's mine returned to me, what's hers returned to her. I felt tingly sensations in my hands, lightheaded at times, and most interestingly, I felt sad. I was mourning. As with any relationship, it wasn't all bad. So to say goodbye wasn't only triumph and vindication. It was also a single tear and a whispered goodbye. We did have good times. I didn't want it to end this way. Be well, get better, you can do it.

"She may contact you or reach out," she says to me.

She did.

At this point, we're only halfway through our session. We addressed four other lifetimes, but I won't tell you in detail about any more of it. You get the idea, and the rest is just for me.

Instead, I'll leave you with the last image I had in the fifth-dimensional space. It's that of Saraswati facing me, taking my head in her hands, tipping our foreheads towards one another, third eye to third eye, in love. Big smiles and an open road.

ANNA LIEBERMAN
~ CONTRIBUTING WRITER ~

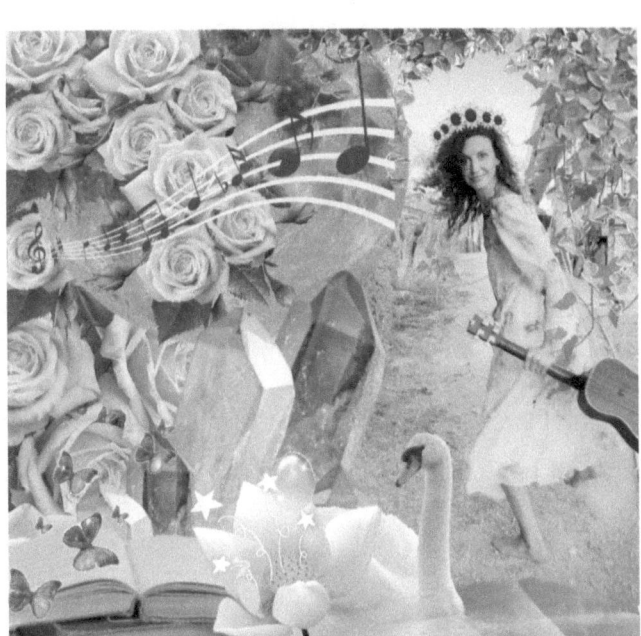

Anna is an artist, actress and writer most known for her lead role in The Best People. She received her B.A. in theatre arts from Westmont College (2009) Shortly after, Anna was cast by Frank Oz in her first television guest star role on Leverage. After a brief stint in T.V, she began working with AFI film conservatory students, where she starred in six short films, including the Student Oscar-winning 'This Way.'

Saying:

"The future of the world depends on the full restoration
of the Sacred Feminine in all its tenderness,
passion, divine ferocity,
and surrendered persistence."

~ Andrew Harvey

CHAPTER 7

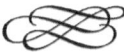

DURGA, MA'AT GODDESS ACTIVATIONS™

Abigail Diaz Juan

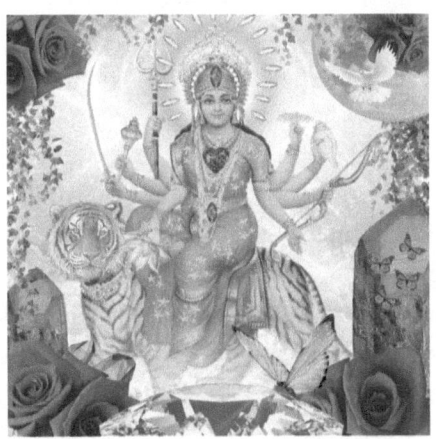

Blooming Laughter

*A*s one of the authors in the Awakening Starseeds book series, I had enjoyed my relationship with Radhaa and her Mother, Maya The Shaman, for a couple of years now, and I was ready for the next phase of my spiritual journey. It was no surprise that Radhaa had gotten a tap on the shoulder by the Universe and just wanted to check in on me, and this led me to book a Goddess Activations™ session soon after. The Goddess couldn't have come at a more pivotal time in my life.

I have been embroiled in a legal issue for several months. The plaintiff, driven by fear and desperation, was ferocious and relentless in her attacks on me, unwarranted as they were.

My opponent was not interested in winning the case, and she was unnaturally obsessed with destroying my companies. A few months back, just after the onset of the lawsuit, in one of my joint meditation sessions where a partner and I travel together up to the "Heart of Creator," which she learned from Maya that the heart of creator is the place to go, to witness each other receive divine information on our destiny work. A woman unexpectedly appeared to both of us in a state of fear and misery. We were able to see the demons that had taken hold of her and were using her as their instrument and medium to annihilate me to prevent me from accomplishing my critical mission on Earth. This was not the first attempt demons have tried to destroy me by any means, but it was their first time using the civil legal system as their arena of choice to do battle.

Her Machiavellian "the ends justify the means" approach taught me that perception was more important than the truth in the legal arena. I had my hands full, piercing through her many illusionary veils of accusations, lies, exaggerations, and hyperbole to get the court to see the real truth at hand. We were now at the discovery stage of the legal process, where we were exchanging heated body blows in hand-to-hand combat of life or death as the plaintiff tried to maneuver me off the edge of a cliff.

No stranger to the battlefield, having been a seasoned warrior in business and a light warrior in Spirit for quite some time, being able to fight from an integrated position of above (unseen) and below (seen) has made me a formidable opponent over the years. When Radhaa appeared, I knew that divine assistance had arrived, and the fight was about to turn in my favor. I responded immediately and scheduled my Goddess Activation™ for the very next day.

That night before the Activation, Radhaa told me to think of the Goddess I wanted to meet. I drew a blank on a particular name, my spiritual discipline/philosophy being more of a Star Trek/Galactic bent than one of the deities, Goddesses, and Gods. Instead, I sensed that there would be more than one Goddess appearing in my session. Who they would be, I hadn't a clue. This was also my first Goddess Activations™ experience, so I had no set expectations.

Monday morning, I woke up with the name of Goddess Lakshmi in my head, so I told Radhaa that she would be appearing. At the onset of the session, when Radhaa took me to my mystical spot, it was Goddess Durga who met me instead.

In Hindu cosmology, Goddess Durga is the Mother of the Universe and is believed to be the power behind creating, preserving, and destroying the world. Considered the fiercest warrior of all Hindu goddesses, she is the staunch protector of the dharma of the light and the good. Goddess Durga appears on the battlefield of spiritual warfare when demonic forces are causing psychic unrest and physical distress within a person.

Goddess Durga revealed that I had already ascended out of what was known in Hinduism as a Yuga cycle in my past lives, an era of 4,320,000 years. She went on to explain that I had volunteered, like many other ascended light beings, to come back into another cycle to assist humanity in its collective transition to the Golden Age of Mankind timeline, making my mission in this incarnation significantly critical in both its purpose and timing.

As regaled in the Mahabharata epic poem, in my previous Yuga Cycle, during the Bhagavad-Gita, Radhaa saw that I was a warrior in the time of Krsna. I was considered a great warrior and general, fighting alongside Krishna in the great galactic battles that ensued. Leading my armies, I had defeated many demonic forces in that war. Then Radhaa saw me moving about the field of battle in my vehicle, a futuristic flying chariot connected to my third eye.

The demons I fought with, because of their base nature, could not ascend on their own. When I returned to Earth, this time, recognizing who I previously was, these earthbound demons began to soul stalk me. I had an innocence, integrity, and energetic lightness of these earthbound demons desired and needed. I was nectar to them. As Goddess Durga recounted this, it began to make sense of all the many incidents of close death encounters, dangerous situations, and attempts to destroy me that I experienced over the years. In overcoming these situations over the past decades, I developed into a seasoned warrior personally and professionally. Today, Durga cleared my third eye to see more clearly any demon coming my way and discern quickly the situations they create.

Then Radhaa took me away from my mystical spot to the great heart of Creator, where I was met by my whole galactic family, guides, angels, and ancestors. It was quite a large congregation. I am humbled and grateful for having such an enormous support team in the higher dimensions, heavenly realms, and divine planes of existence.

The Appearance of Three other Goddesses

Then much to Radhaa's surprise and delight, three additional Goddesses graced us with their presence, Lakshmi, Quan Yin, and Ma'at. There I was, seated in the center with Goddess Durga to my front supporting the warrior in me, Goddess Lakshmi to my back giving me support in abundance, Goddess Quan Yin to my right holding love and compassion; and Goddess Ma'at to my left holding justice.

Radhaa shared with me that this was highly unusual because the Goddess showed themselves all at the same time. Not only was the appearance of Goddess Durga, Mother of the Universe, significant and auspicious enough on its own. "This was probably one of the most intensive and longest sessions with the most Goddesses! It's not usual that there are four! There is usually One per Activation - as the energy is so intense in the presence of ONE benevolent and Ascended being."

I have been suffering from extreme shoulder and upper back pain for the past few weeks ever since we entered the lawsuit's discovery phase and began trading blows. It was so bad that I couldn't sit at the computer for any length of time and had been reduced to mainly sitting in bed propped up with pillows for the past two weeks.

I was under a demonic attack, and that spot between my shoulder blades happened to be a weak spot health-wise, therefore vulnerable to assault. With the other three Goddesses giving support, Durga introduced me to a simple but profound way to heal myself from painful demonic attacks and fight future demonic attempts. In Radhaa's explanation, "Instead of meeting evil and hostility in the 3D with aggression and anger, she introduced me to a form of spiritual love-based aikido that Radhaa described as "blooming laughter."

Goddess Durga brought divine light into my body, first into my womb, where we saw a beautiful green-blue dragonfly that would later appear in the physical realm in front of Radhaa when the Activation concluded. Then Radhaa guided the light towards my right shoulder blade, where my physical pain was the most severe. The light covered the entire area, creating enlightened space between the muscle fibers and my vertebrae.

Next, she had me access a memory filled with laughter in my past where I was most childlike and innocent, totally immersed in solely enjoying life. I drew upon a childhood moment when I was ten years old in Kandahar, Afghanistan, playing in the expatriate community swimming pool together with my friends, with not a care in the world as I dive-bombed into the water, blissfully unaware of what challenges were yet to come in my adulthood. Back then, I didn't know what fear was, surrounded only by freedom and love. Radhaa had me capture that moment in time into a smiley face symbol.

Goddess Durga and Radhaa became one while working on me. She had me superimpose that smiley face onto my painful spot to encircle and enclose the affected area. She then placed a lotus flower atop that smiley face. Within moments, the lotus flower began to bloom. As its petals unfurled, black gunk began to ooze out between the petals as if the flower was drawing out the toxic negativity in my body through that specific spot between my vertebrae and right shoulder blade. As the leaching process continued, more flowers appeared and bloomed, black gunk oozing from their petals. I could feel a reaction of lessening pain accompanying the imagery.

Goddess Durga then began to explain what she was doing to do the procedure independently in the future. I was to incorporate this clearing technique into my daily routine and apply it towards any area of pain in my body for general overall wellness and protection against attacks from dark forces.

Like our individual energy signatures, we are each born with an original blueprint unique to ourselves. As we grow and age, we develop a pain body that overlays that blueprint as we respond to our life experiences and society. Pretty soon, that painful body expands to the point of encompassing who we are and all we know, separating ourselves from our original blueprint, which is absent of any pain, toxicity, and negativity. When we feel pain and discomfort, physically, mentally, or emotionally, we are experiencing our pain body. In contrast, the purity of innocence we each have within our core reconnects us to our original blueprint. To access that original blueprint, we need to remember pain-free memories of innocence, joy, and happiness as they are direct conduits to the natural person we each inherently are. Those memories are more abundant in our childhood, where we are most innocent and unknowing of pain, fear, and darkness.

By superimposing those happy memories (smiley face) on top of the actual pain and discomfort, wherever it exists within our physical, emotional, or mental bodies, we penetrate through to our original blueprint lying underneath our surface pain body. By applying flowers that bloom away from the toxicity of the pain-body layer, we dissolve that area of our pain body, thereby regaining parts of our original blueprint, resulting in us experiencing that original state of natural being once again. Radhaa suggests I do this daily. The more we do this blooming laughter technique, the more we can dissolve areas of our pain body and directly access the underlying aspects of our original blueprint, which is strong, healthy, abundant, prosperous, peaceful, transformative, and resourceful.

Then Goddess Durga turned her attention to the other application of this blooming laughter technique, the application of spiritual aikido against aggression and attack. She had me visualize lining up all my opponents in the lawsuit, from the plaintiff and her opposing counsel to all supporting parties involved that are or could affect me negatively, including the actual lawsuit itself. Next, Goddess Durga had me superimpose that same smiley face onto opponents' line in the lawsuit so that that smiley face fully enclosed them.

Then Radhaa asked me what I saw.

I saw a traditional classroom with a wall of windows on the left. At the front of the room next to the door on the right, was the lawsuit, the plaintiff, her opposing counsel, and the people who were supporting her; in particular, the key player behind the scenes directing the strategy against me whom I had been unaware of until now. They were all lined up shoulder to shoulder, and I could see them from where I sat in the back of the room. We were the only occupants in the room.

Then, I began to see hundreds of rose petals coming through the windows as if carried by the wind, streaming towards the line of people and dropping in piles around their feet. As the petals continued to float towards them, Radhaa increased the flow to "thousands of flowers," and pretty soon, the vertical piles of petals had risen to a height above each person's head, covering them and space between them and me completely in petals. All I could see were mounds of red rose petals everywhere.

After what seemed like a minute of seeing rose petals everywhere, all the petals began to disappear until there was nothing left gradually. Not a single petal in sight nor a single person in front of me. Had the rose petals vanquished the people? I wasn't sure. Nevertheless, I was now alone in the room.

One week later, after my session with Radhaa, when I went back up again in meditation to the heart of the Creator, I saw the lawsuit actively crumble into a pile of rubble before me. The next day, my attorney received a notification email from opposing counsel that they canceled depositions and stepped back due to 'recent developments in the case.

I can only conclude that by vanquishing the demons with the

blooming laughter technique, the plaintiff, when set free from the grip of these demons, realized how self-destructive and costly the path she had gone down in her blind obsession to destroy me. Awakened from her nightmare, her actions no longer made sense when viewed in the stark light of reason. Thankfully, I now sense a quiet silence emanating from the plaintiff, absent of the intense, frenzied aggressive irrational energy that had been previously coming from her and the lawsuit itself.

Goddess Durga finished my session by imparting her essence to call upon her whenever I needed her warrior strength. Goddess Lakshmi, Goddess Quan Yin, and Goddess Ma'at each did the same as well. Radhaa advised me that the codes downloaded during this session from the four goddesses would continue to unpack within me and be cognizant of their effects over the next 30 days.

As Radhaa drew the session to a close, the dragonfly with her iridescent green-blue wings first seen in my womb appeared once again, this time in the physical perched on a leaf before her.

When I looked up "Dragonfly" in my Medicine Cards book authored by Jamie Sams and David Carson, here is what I read:

"Dragonfly…
Breaks illusions,
Brings visions of power,
No need to prove it,
Now is the hour!
Know it, believe it,
Great Spirit intercedes,
Feeding you, bless you,
Filling all your needs."

Abigail Diaz Juan

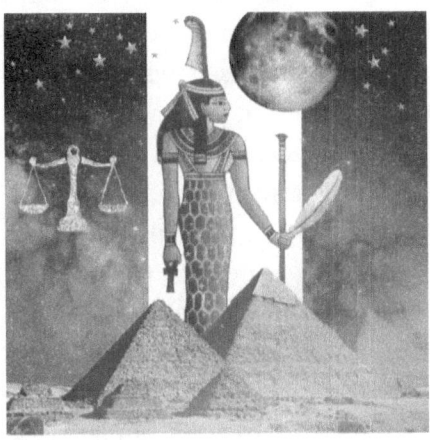

Part Two: Katana of the Divine Feminine
Ma'at, Lakshmi and Quan Yin Goddess Activations™

Continued from Part 1...

*L*egend has it that when a master sword-smith creates a samurai sword in Japan, the steel is tempered and folded a thousand times in the fire before it is deemed worthy of being used. Imbued by the essence of its Creator's spiritual ancestors, a katana of this excellence can take on supernatural prowess, easily obliterating the weaponry of its enemies.

As mentioned in Part 1: Blooming Laughter, I am no stranger to the battlefield, a seasoned business warrior by vocation and light warrior by destiny.

It has been almost a month since my Goddess Activations™ session with Radhaa. As I look back, I can see the profound change within me and the true purpose of the Universe tapping Radhaa on the shoulder, prompting her to connect me to a Goddess Activations™ unexpectedly.

The lawsuit had been like a small landmine in the middle of a road blocking the passage of an entire financial convoy of resources meant to launch my destiny work of working with women entrepreneurs around the world so they could provide help and assistance to their communities. As small in size as it was in magnitude, the lawsuit carried the potential to derail the necessary funding of my project and needed to be neutralized quickly. I am grateful to the Universe for sending me divine support in such a timely manner.

Unfamiliar as I was to working with Goddesses and gods in my spiritual practice, Radhaa suggested I request Maya The Shaman's help working with Goddesses Durga, Lakshmi, Quan Yin, and Ma'at regarding the lawsuit. With Maya the Shaman's facilitation and the Goddesses' assistance and within a week after the Activation, the lawsuit shifted its adversarial posture from an aggressive to a passive stance, allowing my much-needed project funding to move forward unobstructed.

However, that was not all that transpired from my Goddess Activations™ session. As women, we live in a patriarchal society where men define, create, and enforce the sportsmanship rules of conduct, protocol, and competition. This is true in business as well as in our social lives. Men dominate, and to work with them and compete against them, we women must learn how to fight and conduct ourselves according to the male definition of appropriate behavior and successful accomplishment, especially in the business world where power and control are measured by the strength of one's financial means.

As a result, we women become extensions of men because they train us to act and fight as combatants in a competitive battlefield where zero-sum games are fought daily and fear, self-interest, and arrogance reign supreme. I was one of those warriors and even fancied myself a samurai warrior with my own code of honor and superior conduct. The qualities of combat I learned were maneuvers befitting the survival of the fittest in a cutthroat world where the only person who had your back was yourself. Books of power and military strategy such as Sun Tzu's *Art of War,* Niccolò Machiavelli's *The Prince, 48 Laws of Power* by Robert Greene et al., and *On War* by Carl

Philipp Gottfried von Clausewitz, graced the bookshelves of my office.

The only book on my shelf that stood out in stark contrast because a woman wrote it was *The Princessa: Machiavelli for Women* by Harriet Rubin, where she urged one to not just be in men's game but to change the game to a woman's rules of conduct. She taught us how to apply our female attributes as weaponry, yet her advice still mirrored her male counterparts as it was still combative. A different game indeed, but same war.

From this gladiator training, I became adept and seasoned in hand-to-hand combat and excelled in my business endeavors up to a certain point. Acute vigilance, speed, and acumen became qualities necessary for my survival. However, the more I excelled externally, the more alone and miserable I became internally, and the more exhausted I physically became. I became not who I AM as a female, and the constant conflict tore me apart inside. I just ran faster, worked harder, and became more paranoid than my opponents and colleagues.

When the North Star on your compass is set solely on reaching the summit of success, everything falls by the wayside, and your soul gets left behind in your ego's single-minded pursuit of its destination. Pretty soon, you reach a point where you no longer can find your way back home, lost as you are in the weeds of your daily existence.

It took a spontaneous kundalini awakening cloaked in a debilitating illness to catapult me out of that ego-oriented competitive world, sending me on an inner journey of many years to rediscover my soul and reunite me to the spiritual mission I had returned to Earth to do.

From a socio-economic perspective, the biggest issue facing women is isolation, vulnerability, and ignorance, leading to poverty, helplessness, frustration, fear, and loneliness. Separated and isolated from a feminine support network and safety net, a woman or a girl can drown in a sea of ignorance, violence, and abuse, unaware of what she can potentially become, unable to sustain herself and her children; eventually becoming a light snuffed out by the darkness of her circumstances.

Even though we make up half of the world's population, to better understand the gross inequity of women from the perspective of global economics and money flow, imagine a funding pyramid where the base is debt-based (Microfinance), and the tip is investment-based (Venture Capital). The global market for Microfinance which services low-income and the poorest of the poor is projected to reach US$313.7 billion by 2025. In 2018, 80% of microfinance borrowers were female necessity entrepreneurs surviving in a financial arena wherein 2019. It took only 25 billionaires to equal the wealth of the bottom 50% of the world's population. Contrast that with the global Venture industry where only 2.3% of its total raised capital of US$80.7 billion in 2020 went to female-led startup opportunities, a minuscule percentage increase from the mere 2% in funding given to female entrepreneurs back in 2000.

I stand today at the threshold of my new life, fully prepared and finally ready to take on what I incarnated this time to do, the creation of a fourfold integrated structure of incubation, education, investment, and stewardship capable of activating a million points of light out of the darkness within a 100-year timeframe.

The Million Points of Light Initiative is to create a grassroots think tank ecosystem composed of women from communities worldwide that will be global in design and implementation and laterally focused on grassroots community improvement through the worldwide development of women entrepreneurs as next-age CEOs business owners, and community leaders.

A few weeks after Radhaa's Goddess Activations™ session, I finally realized its timely purpose and why these four goddesses showed up in particular. By undertaking a destiny this massive, I needed all the divine assistance I could get.

Our society is so fear-driven that poverty, helplessness, and violence run rampant throughout the world. In this darkness, we females must bring in the light of the Divine Feminine if we are to save humanity from its own Armageddon. And yet, it begs the question of how can we women expect to change the way the game of life is played if we have been trained to act like the very men who have brought humanity to the brink of destruction? As warriors of light, how can women transform society so corrupted by fear, inequity, and divisiveness into an enlightened and evolved society inspired by love, equality, and community?

As a samurai warrior, combatant, and gladiator, I learned from men how to conquer, take and capture market space at the expense of another. Having regained my soul, will I behave differently this time in my re-entry into the business world, or will I revert to my old training in the heat of battle?

Enter the four Goddesses led by Goddess Durga, the great Hindu warrior Goddess and Mother of the Universe. She is legendary for vanquishing vast demonic armies, especially when Kali, the Goddess of destruction, emerges from her forehead to create death and destruction amongst the enemy. Since time immemorial, Goddess Durga has been worshiped as the supreme power (Shakti) of the Supreme Being and revered in many Hindu scriptures.

Even though Goddess Lakshmi is considered a Hindu Goddess, she is also seen as a Universal Goddess of Fortune, bringing wealth, prosperity, abundance, beauty, and love into people's lives when called upon. As each of us goes through our dark night of the soul, Goddess Lakshmi restores balance in all aspects of our lives through universal abundance. She represents beauty, majesty, grace, purity, fertility, wealth, knowledge, and serenity. To respect her is to respect all that is important to me. Abundance and auspiciousness personified; she is the Divine power of success that transforms people's dreams into reality, bringing them both material and spiritual wealth on all levels. Embodying her energy is both a spiritual act and a practical approach in applying ancient wisdom to modern life.

The chief Goddess of all East Asia, Goddess Quan Yin, is the Goddess of compassion and mercy and has often been compared to the Virgin Mary, Mother of Jesus. She personifies harmony, grace, and balance, key attributes of Enlightenment. Goddess Quan Yin is one of the San Ta Shih, the Three Great Beings, renowned for their power over the animal kingdom or the forces of nature. As one of the deities most frequently seen on altars in Chinese temples,

Goddess Quan Yin is the shortened version of "One Who Sees and Hears the Cry from the Human World," meaning she hears our prayers. Goddess Quan Yin especially worshipped by women, comforts the troubled, the sick, the lost, the senile, and the unfortunate. As one of the most beloved Buddhist gods, she is considered the model of great Chinese beauty. Goddess Quan Yin shows us that Enlightenment is attainable, and by choosing compassion over fear, judgment, and anger, we are practicing Enlightenment in the here and now.

Goddess Ma'at is the ancient Egyptian Goddess of truth, order, justice, harmony, and balance. In translation, Ma'at means 'truth' in Egyptian. As one of their most powerful and highly regarded Goddesses, the Egyptians believe that the Universe is an ordered and rational place because of her. From Goddess Ma'at, they understood that everything in the Universe follows a pattern, which the Greeks also referred to as the underlying order of the Universe's logos. The concept of Ma'at is what grounded the reality of the world Egyptians lived in, both morally and physically. Therefore, proper behavior and conduct were determined by Goddess Ma'at. As the karmic judge for the Universe, she created a template of 42 codes of ethics for Egyptian society to live by. When a person dies, their heart is placed on a scale balanced by Goddess Ma'at herself or by the feather of Ma'at to determine if they have followed the practice of Ma'at in their life. If not, their heart is devoured by a demon. If the answer is yes, then they are allowed to pass into the afterlife.

Lightweights by no means, these four legendary 'badass' goddesses appeared at my session, and I sat up and took notice. Radhaa had told me that their essences would integrate within me over the next 30 days, and I had no idea what that meant. As I approach the end of the 30 days since my session with Radhaa, I am beginning to understand the important significance of their appearance.

I committed to Radhaa to write about my Goddess Activations™ experience for her new book within two weeks of my session. To my distress, I drew a blank each time I sat down to write, and the words just refused to flow. Thankfully, Radhaa understood and extended my deadline. I went up with my meditation partner to the heart of Creator to find out why I had such writer's block.

We found ourselves facing a Parthenon-shaped open-air temple. Then one by one, each of the four goddesses appeared before us, playfully arrayed amongst the Greek temple's columns. Then the temple's Doric columns dissolved into pillars of light, and I heard the goddesses address my concern of regressing to my combative way of doing business as I began working on the Million Points of Light Initiative. As they embody the Divine Feminine within me, I too embody the Divine Feminine within them. By embedding their combined essences into me in the form of the Divine Feminine goddess archetype, I can draw upon their supernatural qualities, gifts, and wisdom at any time. Divine Feminine personified, I will gracefully re-enter the business world assured and sure-footed in my femininity.

The temple disappeared, but Goddesses Durga, Lakshmi, Quan Yin, and Ma'at remained. Other Goddesses appeared around them until a sea of goddesses stood shoulder to shoulder, hundreds of rows deep before us. Then they all began to hum in unison until the sound "Om" built to a thunderous roar in our ears. This went on for several minutes until gradually, the hum lowered to a whisper and then stopped. Having attuned us with their blessing, the deities slowly disappeared until there were just the two of us left staring at each other awestruck at what we had just witnessed and received.

The Oxford Dictionary defines "tempered" as The origin of the old English word "temprian" is to 'bring something into the required condition by mixing it with something else. As a verb, it improves the hardness and elasticity of metal by reheating and cooling it; or acting as a neutralizing or counterbalancing force (something). The noun originally denoted a proportionate mixture of elements or qualities. Also, the combination of the four bodily senses of humor believed in medieval times to be the basis of [one's] temperament.

As a katana of the Divine Feminine, now imbued with the proper temperament to fight on her behalf, I humbly thank my four goddess archetypes. From Goddess Durga, my warrior nature is now tempered with tenderness and love. From Goddess Quan Yin, compassion and mercy will always guide my actions. From Goddess Lakshmi, wisdom and generosity of Spirit now dictate my choices. And from Goddess Ma'at, I will conduct myself with fairness, justice, and balance, in harmony always with the Universe.

Later that day, I sat down at my computer, and the words of this story came pouring out of my fingertips onto the keyboard.

Salamat Po.

Abby

ABIGAIL DIAZ JUAN
~ CONTRIBUTING WRITER ~

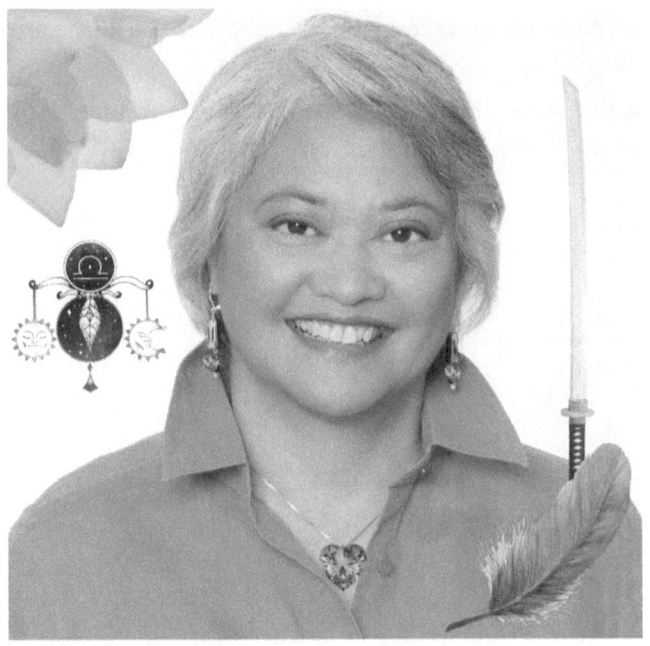

Years ago, **Abigail Diaz Juan** reached her pinnacle of business success as a Venture Capitalist, managing her very own multi-billion-dollar venture fund in Silicon Valley. Her experience in the world of business incubation, entrepreneurism, and high finance made her realize the enormous imbalance in how little funding and support women entrepreneurs received in contrast to their male counterparts.

When her destiny came knocking, it triggered a spontaneous kundalini awakening disguised as a debilitating illness, forcing her to retire from that successful life to prepare her for what she would become today, a champion for women entrepreneurs.

Back from her intense spiritual journey of many years, Abigail Diaz Juan stands poised to re-enter the international business arena to balance the scales of inequity through the development of a global program called "The Million Points of Light Initiative," which will provide much-needed funds, tools, and resources to help women entrepreneurs become inspired leaders and successful business owners in their own right.

An international speaker, venture capitalist, spiritual entrepreneur, women's empowerment advocate, and author of "How Me Found I: Mastering the Art of Pivoting Gracefully Through Life," Abby can be reached at: www.AbigailDiazJuan.com

CHAPTER 8

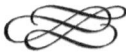

SOPHIA GODDESS ACTIVATIONS™

Alanna Starr

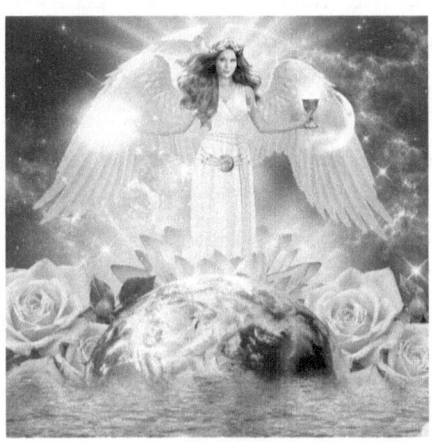

A Divine Invitation

"I am an endless uncurling rose guided by the Spirit of Truth."

*C*an humanity feel the Hand of the Mother at work? It's crazy to think that in 2021, many still have no understanding of the importance and relevance of the Divine Feminine or the Great Goddess. It is why the Pillars of Light Goddess Activations™ experience is powerful for women like me who see the significance of this Sacred Work.

It is the Holy Mother of All Life, In the name of Goddess Sophia, that I called upon to activate me deeper into the sacred mysteries. There are countless ways to describe who and what Sophia is. In short, she is known as Divine Wisdom in Greek, intelligence, and cleverness. Wisdom has guided every other Goddess and Ascended Master throughout ages and generations. She is behind the "fallen Goddess" scenario, and some would argue that she's the force behind Taoist "The Way," King Solomon's Wisdom, and Jesus and Mary Magdalene's teachings.

Sophia is Gaia, and Gaia is Sophia - ultimately, Sophia is the Wisdom of the Earth and Mother of All Living. She descends and ascends from Heaven to Earth, animating all the elements. She is the feminine principle of the God-Head and Chokmah on the Kabbalah Tree of Life. Sophia is divine insight, pure inspiration, and a deep inner-knowing at the very core. Of course, this is all up for interpretation based on each individual's experience with the Divine Sophia. There is much to discover, and while I have learned a great deal in my studies, I know the value of one's journey of researching Who and What Sophia is to them. She awaits her children to seek her, know her, and be filled with her Holy Spirit.

A Significant Friendship

I've known Radhaa for over seven years, and we've always had a close sisterhood connection and shared deep conversations. It was all meant to be this way to get me to see how magical the dots connected up to this point. It's obvious. Sophia knows I needed this synchronicity to step into my voice as an author in this chapter. As I wrote this, I decided to research the word "synchrony," To my surprise, it comes from the Greek word "Sunkhronos," meaning: Together with/in time. Understanding "the time is now" or "your time is at hand" came to me from previous synchronicities. Sophia does this beautiful spiritual symbolism in which the mystical synchronicity follows like the shadow gently nudging us towards experiences that activate us into higher vibrations. That's what Radhaa's session has exactly given me and more mystical proof of the behind-the-scenes workings of the Great Mother Goddess. Once again, I'm inspired to share this Wisdom in writing, teaching, creating art, sharing, and being authentically me.

I knew about Radhaa's Goddess Activations™ healings but hadn't experienced a session personally until Pillars of Light came to be. Goddess Activations is truly a magical healing modality designed to empower and up-level your soul at a galactic level. Every time I listen to the recording of our session, I go back into a trance state because it was so powerful. If you ever get the chance to work with Radhaa, you're in for an insightful experience. Even if you've been on the awakened journey, there may be more waiting to be discovered. Radhaa's medicine is calming, allowing a wealth of akashic goodies to come through.

The invitation to receive Goddess Activations™ came as a symbol of answered prayers for clarity and further initiation. It's a cosmic call to share sacred responsibility as an activated Goddess across all time and space. When I received the message from Radhaa to become a "Pillar of Light" to share my Goddess Activations™ story as a contributing writer for the Goddess, my in-divine-flow meter went off like crazy. I thought to myself: "Yes! I want to be a Pillar of Light! I want to be a living embodiment of the Goddess." This title is also an undeniable quest I enjoy taking. I knew that all the work done in the name of the Goddess had come to a culmination after my session with Radhaa. This chapter symbolically represents my spiritual graduation and signifies a time of transformation as I embody more of the light of my soul.

The ironic thing is that although I have this longing to represent the Holy Mother in this way, now and then, nagging insecurities pop in to wreak havoc and distract me from my path. The distractions have come in different forms and disguises throughout my life placed within me purposely through negative agendas and accidentally. Just because you know how "life happens," doesn't mean you know it all. After having my first child five months ago during the Covid19 pandemic, I felt out of alignment with my spiritual work. This session gave me clarity once again to restore order in my temple, refocus my energy and recalibrate my spiritual path. Since then, I've regained a more certain and profound belief in my mission, passion, and calling without the same old stories and attachments. Sophia's love emanates from all directions, and with this integration of mind, body, and soul, my Heaven on Earth blueprint feels more restored, and I'm ready to burst with joy! Hallelujah!

Hunter of Vision

In the past, I've been called the "Midwife of the New Paradigm" by those who can see me beyond my insecurities and understand what my role here is as a way-shower. When I heard this name, it resonated with me because there is a global rebirth taking place, and it's a blessing to hold the codes for the awakening of Heaven on Earth. Doing healing is important because we often can't get out of our suffering, which is a big soul trap. Many believe we are headed into the Golden Age, while others would assume the darkest days are ahead--either way, this is a time of utmost importance. Each of us must choose the path we want to dwell in: to activate Goddess Codes™ that awaken us to Divine Love as her children or remain an orphaned victim of the illusion of separation. Understanding the Divine Feminine is the catalyst for this cosmic remembrance and outpouring of light codes coming into the earth at this time. It's the Goddess pouring her Wisdom on those who have eyes to see and ears to hear. My channels are now open and receptive while making me a target to the opposing forces like a fly buzzing toward the light. "Stand in the light of your soul," Sophia proclaimers instill over and over again.

There was a point in the session where I went from "Radhaa has known me for so long, she will already know what to say to me... how will I know if it's Sophia?" to "oh my Goddess, without a doubt, this is real! Of course, this is Sophia speaking--this is happening!" Sophia spoke precisely to me through Radhaa using words and different personal symbology that felt aligned with her as I know her. Don't get me wrong--I completely believe people can channel. It's just that with all the belief of her I hold so dear, there was still this doubt and confusion embedded in me from timelines of separation. Radhaa called in my Higher Self, and the doubt began to dissipate. While there was some tightness and anxiety, there was a feeling of euphoria and an electric tingling through the center of my body. As soon as Sophia made her presence known, crystalline codes rushed into my crown chakra. I recall visualizing beautiful crystals shimmering in a pearlescent luminous light, and it was a grand feeling.

I receive this session from Radhaa because I have numerous gifts and crystalline star codes that my divine higher self urges me to share to express here on earth. I realized that it's safe for me to be seen in my power to do these powerful things. I remember Sophia asked me to give up my burdens to her in exchange for more light of my soul and higher self to come through. My divine higher self was in communion with Sophia, and they both made it clear to me that I won't need to question what is coming to me anymore because I will know it will be pure communication and channeling. My higher self was catching up to my lower self, closing the gaps and in between, no longer making me resistant to the downloads coming to me.

> Could you do me a favor?
> Don't even look at me for who I tell you I am
> Don't believe a word.
> Nothing that you've heard
> Until you've experienced my truth
> Could you do me a favor and look at me through the?

> Eyes of a thousand suns
> Look at me through the eyes of above.
> Return to Innocence

Sophia lovingly reminds me that "my holiness and purity can never be taken away." We forget because of the pain this world can cause us. Walking with the Goddess can give us the gift of understanding, redemption, and resurrection to see us through suffering. On my journey, I have been linked to countless others who've walked the path of The Goddess. This path led me long ago to meet Radhaa at a "Goddess Gathering" Facebook group filled with women all over the globe who felt the same calling. Many of us women led in the Divine Feminine direction have endured immense pain and trauma in which we consciously turned into Wisdom. We all have come to meet an aspect of the Goddess through transmutation and alchemical transformation. Through heart intelligence, we can transcend into higher frequencies of love, forgiveness, mercy, and compassion- these are some of the teachings of the Goddess.

My childhood was not easy. When Radhaa and Sophia had me tap into my inner child, it brought to my attention that I still had core wounds that needed care, compassion, and release. I could not deny this was the case, especially after admitting that my dreams had been traumatic and torturous the past few months. It was literally as if my biggest fears in Dreamtime were torturing me. It was clear there was a gap between my spirit and my physical body and that I was being blocked. As blockages got cleared, my sleep became better, and my dreams were not as scary.

Sophia speaks to my heart with a remembrance of my pure, holy innocence. We are Holy. We are Pure! She says to me many times in my session that all I have suffered was part of the divine plan. In all my meditative experiences, Sophia reminds me of this, but in this experience, she is saying, "enough is enough." No more hiding in the shadows--as a pillar of light, I no longer need to carry these painful memories. I saw myself shedding old limiting beliefs and sadness as she asked me to replace these with memories of happy childhood moments. Times where I felt most connected to her and in love with life- those are things she's wanted me to get in touch with. I now am safe to feel a constant bliss from receiving her love and support. She reminds me that I am worthy of being her disciple. She gave Radhaa a metaphor of filing all those less than happy memories into filing cabinets because she knows that I like things to be organized. Sophia knows my heart's desires and how to soothe me. All I must do is ask for her, and she will show up.

As a child, I didn't feel safe. I always learned boundaries by trial and error because I moved so fast. Sophia asked me to forgive myself for ever feeling less than loved or less than worthy. It's so clear to me now that this is all I have ever wanted was to be a voice of Wisdom and feel safe speaking on behalf of her. My purpose is to share my voice in all ways possible and remind others of their holy divine innocence that "it can never be taken away." It is mine by divine right, and because other powers try to claim dominion over me and what's mine, I must constantly command my divinity and sovereignty.

> See from the sights below.
> Could you think of me Cosmically?
> Feel me Organically
> Divine Sovereignty
> Delightfully and Intentionally
> Care for me, willing.
> When you see me, hug me.

Moving Energy

After tackling the darker energies that were still swirling around, creating blockages and disorder, we activated more of my crystalline christ light, and more unraveling came to me. Radhaa cleared away all the black goo that coated my aura. It was fun to witness Radhaa laughing at the downloads that she was getting from Sophia. She had quite a sense of humor. Sophia and my higher self wanted to clear artificial barricades and holographic images around me in the session.

There was a feeling of fear and distrust about moving into my full power and my true purpose and path. Radhaa conveyed as she has in the past just how big and important my purpose is and that it's very big. A feeling of angst arose as Radhaa began to bring forth what energy and off-planet entities were attached to me throughout my lifetimes. Sophia began to bring in the white flame placed across my chest and began to burn up all artificial technologies and implants. I began to breathe deeply in and out the stuck energies. Sophia placed the white flame and a pillar throughout the core of my body. The white flame melted away all the negativity, clearing a pathway for codes to come through. She brilliantly sent downlight to me and showed us a helmet that blocked my crown chakra from receiving more of my higher self and downloads of information that wanted to come. Sophia illuminated gaps between my multiple bodies. Radhaa called forth my inner child Alanna. She wanted to integrate some healing, and Radhaa lovingly also called back my soul fragments and restored my integrity. Since then, I've been continually filling myself up with her grace and golden bliss as I feel lighter and freer to be me. No longer living in the shadows of all the great Sophia Scholars before me. I am equal, one of her divine sparks. I am truly her humble Priestess.

> Meaningfully
> Wonder deeply and Soulfully
> When you look into my eyes
> See not a disguise
> Could you do your best to help me realize?
> I am I, and You are You

A Stream of a Thousand Roses

Radhaa reminded me through Sophia that I hold the Codes of the Rose within me as she called upon the sacred rose to bloom open at any time. Radhaa's blooming rose healing modality truly was a sign of Sophia's presence. She proclaimed to me that the rose was my secret power. I remember the vivid visualization of the stream of a thousand roses that came from the Heavens and into my crown chakra. I knew for certain that was a sacred gift from her as I recalled a Keycode activation from Ascended Master Mother Mary: "She of a thousand Rose's" in Kai Ra's book, The Sophia Code. Mother Mary is a mentor for "fulfilling your prophecy and the teachings of the rose: the spiral path to open your sacred heart." Mary Magdalene came in strong with her full support and her army of angels. I saw myself standing before Sophia in the ceremony with an open heart allowing the Wise Dakini to awaken within me. Radhaa poured roses into my heart and bloomed wide open, helping me reclaim my sovereignty as a gifted healer. She gave me the gift of the laughing Buddha face--and these are not metaphors but actual gifts of healing. There were a few things for clearing I was asked to recite. I was also given the 30-day protection prayer by Radhaa, a narcissist removal clearing, and a daily mudra called "Kashyapa" to create a protective shell that blocks negative energy. I'm integrating these practices into my life and can see a subtle difference in my energy field.

> Together we make up God's view.
> Universal Factor
> Be Present with Me
> Not a reactor
> Do Us a favor and see me through.
> The eyes of Creator
> Without a single judgment

The Birth of a Mother

Let us consider a mother's love for her child when we ponder what the Goddess Sophia means to us. When I welcomed my first child into the world, it was my greatest accomplishment ever. I realized the most important part of my existence was becoming a mother because I knew it was my destiny. My job as a parent is to protect and preserve the original thought within the being of my children so that they can realize their true GOD reality. To honor the purity and innocence of a child is the most purposeful honor. I can see that it must be similar to Sophia's love for us all, as she's so patient and nurturing while we wake up to remember we are all co-creators in her dream. As I return to my child-like wonder and hold that frequency of compassion and love, I make myself a fantastic mother to my children as Sophia is to us. Motherhood is so much more than the physical birthing of children. It is a way of life.

Bloom

By the end of my session, I couldn't tell who was speaking to me anymore. It was inspiring because I have longed for the open direct dialogue with Sophia. Seeing how Radhaa connected with her on my behalf gave me the courage to believe in myself to do the same for others and trust when Sophia is communicating with me. There truly is a reason for everything--there is nothing our Heavenly Mother does not know. Ultimately, I learned that everything happens for me, not me, and that there's always a divine plan behind the scenes. Thinking this way does not make me naive--it makes me immune to deception. It keeps me grounded and conscious. Knowing this gives me the courage to bloom open at my own pace like a baby rosebud.

What an exciting time to be alive activated as a Goddess walking this earth. I feel a cosmic purpose, and this Goddess Activations™ session with Radhaa helped solidify and amplify these truths that I hold so dear. For this, I am forever grateful. I know for certain that Sophia, the Holy Mother of All Life, is my forever companion. Sophia is rooted in my essence as I am an extension of her. There is power when one stays pure and original to inward knowing of truth, service, non-manipulation, compassion, understanding, and above all else following our "North Star" - our mission. There's more than enough love inside me to mother me and others back into ourselves, just as Sophia does for me. I trust the mother's love that I long for and will use this Wisdom as a flaming torch. You can't gain this experience in a classroom, and it's not found in a degree. It knows my true power--the innate guidance within me that led me into this experience to become a Pillar of Light.

In closing this chapter, I declare and fully accept the Heaven on Earth blueprint within me. The Wisdom of the Goddess has aligned me to a sacred mission to tell the world that She has come and is here. I help set the tone for the feminine archetype as a living embodiment of the Goddess Code™ to heal and inspire. It's a big deal to make this claim, but I would be living a lie if I didn't. Having the light of Sophia and my oversoul means that I can trust the insights that come through and follow my first instinct. I won't question myself so much--the confusion and doubt implants are no more. Out of Samsara and into Satori. If you ever find yourself questioning your value in the world, know that there's a Divine Love that sees you and awaits to be discovered. In the light of three thousand words, thank you, Radhaa, for speaking to me through Sophia, thank you, Sophia, for speaking to me through Radhaa.

We'll be each other's Savior
-Alanna Starr Shimel

Saying:

"There is a collective force rising up on the earth today, an energy of the reborn feminine... This is a time of monumental shift, from the male dominance of human consciousness back to a balanced relationship between masculine and feminine."

~ Marianne Williamson

ALANNA STARR SHIMEL
~ CONTRIBUTING WRITER ~

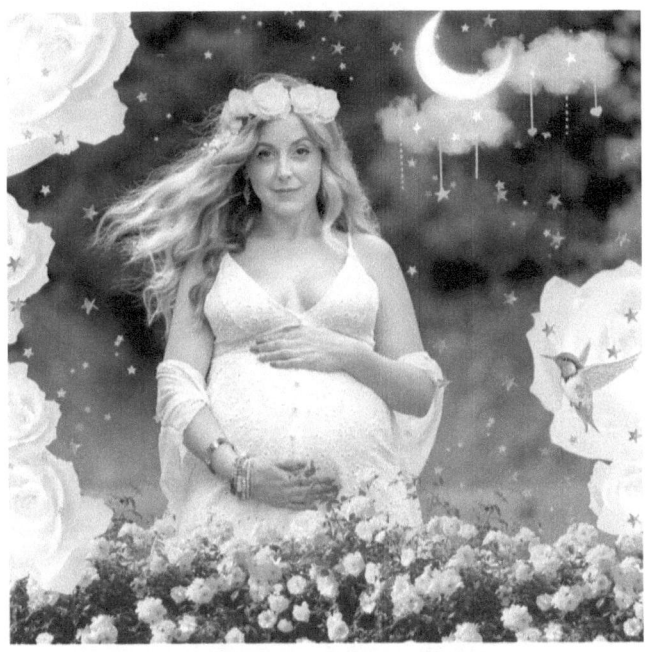

Alanna Starr Shimel is a Mother, Certified Clinical Hypnotherapist, Sacred Song Carrier, Dance Teacher, Researcher, Writer, and Wisdom Keeper dedicated to empowering others on their healing journey through integrating sacred music, insightful Wisdom, and Sacred Knowledge. She is the Creator of "EarthDNA" dried flower forever art and the Curator of Dancenosis, a Mindfulness gnosis dance concept.

Alanna graduated with Honors from Hypnosis Motivation Institute-College Of Hypnotherapy, holds certificates in Past-Life Regression, Handwriting Analysis, and Emotional Freedom Technique, and trained in Red Tent/Women's Mysteries. She keeps a current practice of various energy healing modalities focused on mending the gap between illnesses and the mind & body connection. Her true passions are healing through dance, sound, writing, and helping others return to their divinity. www.alannastarr.com

CHAPTER 9

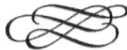

IXCHEL GODDESS ACTIVATIONS™

Raziel F. Arcega

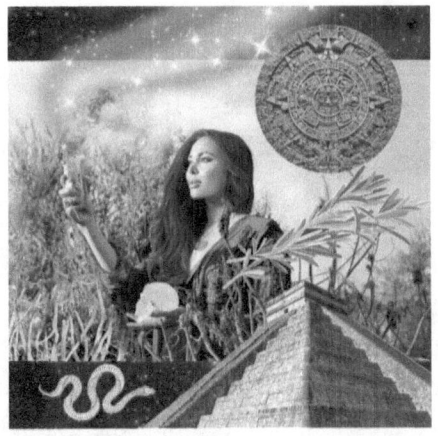

Tuning Into Goddess Ixchel

Time for Activations and it was just one of those days I felt drained, and it felt like it was time to get ready for another phase. I was having this uneasy feeling that I was about to leap into another level in this lifetime, just like a snake about to shed another layer of skin or a butterfly coming out of its cocoon. There was something I wanted to get rid of. Something tells me this is another one of those times for expansion. I have had energy healing sessions on and off for about eight years now, and every time I had a session, it released so much more of the "baggage" that we sometimes could not get rid of ourselves. So we need someone like Radhaa, an energy healer, to bring out what I call the "guck," gooey stuck energies, which are deep-rooted blockages in our energy centers within our body. She could also bring back some of our soul fragments together and let the experience be transformative and energetically rejuvenating, depending on how ready you are to receive. At this point, I knew it was about time.

I knew very little about the full range of Goddess archetypes. Although I was familiar with Mother Mary and Mary Magdalene from Catholic, Aphrodite from Greek Mythology, and Quan Yin from our last Goddess code activation classes I had with Radhaa, there are some real badass Goddesses, and I wanted to pick one who will resonate and work with me and bring out the healing warrior spirit within. I drew some Goddess cards out from a deck I already had and picked out Sekhmet, one powerful Goddess, but Radhaa told me to sit with her for a few days to see and feel a strong connection, but somehow, I wasn't fully connecting with her.

I drew cards again a few times, and Ixchel came out several times, and when I told Radhaa, she was thrilled about it knowing she was a great one. I know little about her, but I got excited too. The first thing that came to mind was another coincidence, I was named Raziel, but my family lovingly called me "Chel" ever since I was a toddler. I don't know what the connection will be, but there might be something there, and I'm willing to explore. Synchronicity and flow are how I lead my life nowadays. Radhaa had mentioned Ixchel was a Mayan Goddess and a very well-known healer at that time. I became more excited and interested in our lineage. I'm from the Philippines, and there is some ancient connection there for sure. Knowing she is Lemurian, that made it so much better. I researched the internet and read up on her, and the more I learned, the more I got thrilled. Goddess Ixchel was a force to be reckoned with.

The Goddess Activations™ & Healing

The day we scheduled the activation, everything in my calendar cleared during the session time for some reason. It was meant to be. Radhaa and I knew that the dark forces are not thrilled when light beings come together, so we had to deal with technical issues that we might have to reschedule, but we pushed through. We eventually connected through zoom, and we started by talking about Ixchel and what she would bring about in our session. I wanted to know more about myself and what keeps me from fully fulfilling my life purpose, and why, for some reason, relationships and money have been a constant issue. I knew some karmic issues and deeper layers that I couldn't tap into on my own. I can pray all I want, but without energetically getting to the root cause or tapping into the subconscious, I will not be able to uncover it nor deal with it. I knew I had to go through another layer of healing so that I can fully be me, be more aware of my life purpose, reclaim my strength and power, cut karmic ties and old bondages that I don't even know nor recall, and to clear out all the negative energies. I have no intention of passing any of it on to my future generations.

Radhaa started the session with her gentleness and protective prayers, and she asked me to settle into a comfortable position. I chose to lie down because I knew how powerful these sessions could be, and I knew I was up for a huge clearing, massive downloads, and transformation. She went into her invocation and chants, and soon enough, I could already feel the energy building up in my body; my right arm started to move faster and faster as she was narrating what she was seeing, where we were, and who was in her presence. She called forth Goddess Ixchel, all the ancestors, ancient ones, spirit guides, guardian angels, and they all came forth. I had my eyes closed, and it felt like I was in a dream state. My body became lighter and lighter. Radhaa was telling me situations and past lives I've had. I went through a life of being an indigenous medicine woman, herbalist, a nun, a shamanic priestess, a slave, and another one where I was of royalty.

Past Life #1:
Disembodied Power within a Relationship

As I laid still, she continued working on my energy to go deeper. Then I started to see I had lost all my possessions because of men or family members who wanted to shut me off from my truth. It wasn't sequential, but we both saw how I was married to a man who enslaved me, took everything I had, including my dignity and who I was meant to be - an abundant light being and a healer. He made me lose my confidence, myself, and power, and I never recovered from that. Perhaps that was why I grew up extremely shy, always wanting to be in the background, and I always felt subservient, not enough, unable to be on my own. It was eye-opening and a relief that now I can deal with this more deeply. At one point, I had lived through a life where there was a romance that included the death of a baby that made me eventually give up hope and was deeply heartbroken. That made me think about relationships I had that turned out to be meaningless and misguided, with trust issues, longing for a partner who would eventually love me for who I truly am. Still, it always turned out they wanted more from me, my money, or my body. When I saw the cycle, I had to stop being in relationships and went on a journey to find myself in the process. I'm glad this is coming forth, surfacing now at the time when I recognize I had more in me that I can't seem to tap into fully. It felt like I was hidden in the abyss or down far below the surface of the Earth. That's how far from my true self I was. I knew a light beaming from within, and the divine spiritual support was so immense, which made me feel so relieved. It was time to unleash me!

Past Life #2: Indigenous Medicine Woman

Radhaa shared my few past lives that came up. We both saw them at the same time. They were all important and especially important in pulling up blockages and healing some aspects of my lost Soul.

Radhaa tuned in and told me she saw me as a young beautiful indigenous woman living in the Philippines. I lived in the mountains, close to a river, and I was wearing indigenous woven outfits and long black hair. As she went deeper, she saw that I was being trained to be a medicine woman at a young age from my mother in this lifetime and my female elders. I was helping women with childbirth, creating holistic remedies, and traditional medicine with herbs.

In the Philippines, so long ago, we had authentic indigenous Shamans, a natural part of this culture before colonization. But at present, Shamans were no longer known. Even though I grew up surrounded by a family in Western medicine, I have always wanted to get into alternative healing modalities, holistic nutrition, and natural plant medicine. I want to bring healing to people through discovering natural foods from the Earth, herbal supplementation, the ancient art of healing through vibrations and energy. She mentioned that she saw me using leaves over people. Clearing their aura and their energetic field like shamanic energy healing. It was a very peaceful life and very connected to nature. I felt one with Earth, my tribe, and my work in that lifetime. I felt this inner knowing deep in my Soul.

Radhaa continued to relate that she saw me when the Spaniards conquered the Philippines, and I felt this terror came over me. They had come to our village, and they had shut down the way we were living, and they took over. Forcing us to become like them and to forget who we were and what our indigenous culture was. I was so hurt and betrayed in that lifetime.

I felt destroyed and pulled away from my gifts, beloved, and life as I knew it. I was taken by one of the Spanish men, a conquistador, who came in with the name of God. This man was a priest, and he forced me to be his wife. He domesticated me, made me wear Spanish clothes, and turned me into a different woman even though I could not understand him. He was so forceful in his ways. I was completely cut off from our own culture and lineage, and this caused an inner death inside of me where I felt so depressed and hopeless. I had lost all my connection to God and the divine Source. I felt that experience cut me off from my divine essence after that lifetime. Radhaa had seen how all these lifetimes became a little heavier on my Soul, and she mentioned it was time for me to reclaim my ancient gifts. To release the shackles of the past and to rise within my intuition. Radhaa explained it in a way my Soul understood.

She told me I was born again as a Filipino in this lifetime because I needed to integrate and come to terms with some aspects of my life as this beautiful indigenous medicine woman. There's outcast energy. A part of me rejects it because I don't think anybody would like me nor understand me, or I would feel like I'd be too weird that I would be an outcast if I practice my indigenous gifts of healing. And so, the outcast energy blocks my blessings. It's blocking my abundance. It's blocking my ability to manifest because there's a part of me that I'm hiding. That's my light. Radhaa said Ixchel asked her to work with me to reconnect and bring back the pieces of me that I had forgotten. It was all taken from me. Stolen. I had to leave behind all my indigenous ways because of emotional trauma. She said I was blocked in expressing this part of me, but it's time to go ahead and reclaim all of it. To own my truth, my gifts, and my ancient heritage.

She reconfirmed that I want to create abundance, create all these things, and be aligned with it. Radhaa reaffirmed and said, "you would be more abundant than you can ever imagine. But you have to step into your truth." And so that's where Ixchel is going to work through Radhaa on this day. Radhaa repeated, "You need to feel safe in your truth because you were abducted from your tribe." I was held captive and not seen, so I am now ready for Ixchel and Radhaa to restore my integrity, my truth, and the authentic code I was gifted with from my original soul blueprint. I am ready for Radhaa to activate my Goddess Code within me. In this session, we're going to work on clearing some of these traumas.

Radhaa observed that I don't like to own my power because I felt it would be taken away once again if I stepped into it. So I would rather be playing small and make many excuses that I'm not good enough! I had to deal with many lifetimes of indoctrinations, and many times I've been pulled away from my true power.

What came up working with Radhaa and Ixchel was my ancient priestess and medicine woman archetype, another lifetime in the Philippines. I was not aligning with my Soul's voice because I was so afraid of being sabotaged again. There's a subconscious fear that if I step into my power, it will repeat the cycle. So it's better not to step fully.

Ixchel says, "Please be kind and loving to yourself. You've been through so much. Your Soul wants this healing, and you have been resisting, because you know that you're very powerful, and you know that this would activate that power within you."

In the meantime, our phone connection got cut off. Radha said there were already interferences in the ethers, negative ones, trying to prevent releasing lifetimes of ownership to my Soul. Radhaa tried to call me back several times, and it was quite a drama of trying to reach me. Finally, when Radhaa did, Ixchel already was in my field wanting to work with me, but I haven't let her in fully yet because I didn't know how powerful this session would be! I tuned in, and I wanted to be that medicine woman. Radhaa said it's coming. There's a lot of people that need my help. I'm stepping into my soul purpose because my purpose was to help people. She said I had been resisting her because I knew my full power was coming back to me.

It's funny because she said I kept saying NO. I said I might not be ready for this, but she's saying I'm just so guarded. So Radhaa held a sacred space for my family tribe healing. In the invocation, we included my lineage, mother, father, etc. Radhaa called out my full name, Raziel Marie Roselyn Fuentebella Arcega, to bring it to the light of clearing and healing. And so it is. I found it so interesting how that all resonates somehow and settles my questions. It gave me the chills. I felt pieces of my Soul come back to me. I felt knowing that I would move forward with my holistic side. I've always had this natural ability to heal myself.

I told Radhaa I once wanted to be a doctor but did not know what type, and since I was told I couldn't handle blood when I was young, a surgeon for sure is not an option. Eventually, I put this career path aside since I could not decide what type of doctor I would be and couldn't even remember my ancient healing roots. Yet, later on, I preferably wanted to be a pediatrician since I love children and am good with them. Ixchel said that I have healing energy inside me, and I'm already accessing it more. That's why I look so young. It brings me to appreciate my lost abilities.

Past Life #3
Clearing Nun-Programming

Radhaa and I also discussed another lifetime where I was a very intuitive type of girl but subservient. I was in Europe somewhere. I have not accepted how my parents in this lifetime wanted me to be. In that previous life, I came from an upper-class family, and they wanted me to go to school and do this or that without regard to what I wanted. They wanted me to be the perfect girl, but the problem was, they also shut me down from my gifts. I was told that I was born a sinner in that lifetime, but they imbued it in me, and I became a nun, more trauma. Radha and I felt that there was a romance there, the death of a baby, and there were a lot of secrets and sadness, sorrow and grief. I felt like I didn't have a choice, and I gave my life up. I did ask God why? I thought about poverty in that lifetime, even though I came from a very rich family. Even though I was from an upper-class family, in some sense, I feel like I'm also a part of the lower class. In another timeline, I've been a servant. In one of my past healings, I remember I was captured as a slave, and I saw myself handcuffed, bound with a rope that I eventually broke free from during the healing sessions I had in this life. These timelines coincide with one another, I always wanted to be a good girl, so I ended up doing just that. But I was very angry and upset and bitter and hurt, and my heart was broken and shattered from losing my baby or had to give it away in that lifetime. I couldn't keep the baby. The disconnect between God-Source and the divine Goddess somehow drained the sense of shame, secrecy, and anguish. It was a very difficult life. I know I needed this part of me to be completely healed.

Final Healing with Radhaa

Radhaa continued to facilitate my healing process and let me know that Ixchel was performing throughout my whole body - sweeping old karmic energies, energetic divorce, infusing light into my root chakra, solar plexus, my heart, and throughout my entire body. I immediately felt like everything was being lifted out of me, and soon after, I told her I felt like crying. Even before I finished the sentence, I cried uncontrollably sobbing and was eventually bawling as if I had held these emotions for centuries, and now the floodgates had just opened. It was tears of relief and of gratitude, of finally being released from multiple lifelong bonds. It was as if my past self was thanking Ixchel for all these releases, for taking me out of my prison, for lifting the curse, for taking the binds off my hands. I was finally at peace. Goddess Ixchel took some time to remove cords and work on my root chakra, where most of the energy and healing needed to occur. I felt much lighter and more relieved afterward. It took us quite a while, and I felt like I went through different lifetimes. I felt the enormous energy of Ixchel. She was a huge figure, very strong, very knowledgeable, and respected by her community. She is quite a Goddess healer, and she was relentless in eliminating everything attached to me. However, she was very gentle and loving in her approach. I thank her for her presence and Radhaa for calling all my ancestors and beings of light to be with me during this activation. Radhaa mentioned that Ixchel would continue to work with me even after the session and help me clear out more karmic energies. I am so grateful to Goddess Ixchel and having Radhaa as a conduit to have this incredible support. I know that in this lifetime, I will clear my karma with the grace of Goddess Ixchel. Does this mean I'm now a badass?

Saying:

"Embracing our divine feminine also means honoring our sacred relationship with the divine instead of seeking validation through institutions. Through the colonial reality, we have been taught that Spirit is something outside of us, something that we need to connect to through an institution, and that must be validated by an authority. Amongst Indigenous cultures, we do not see Spirit as a "field," or as a connection that we must "earn." Instead, we understand that we are an extension of Spirit, that everything is Spirit, and that we are meant to exist in harmony and balance. Embracing our divine feminine allows us to co-create with Spirit and the new world we are seeking."

~ *Dr. Rocío Rosales Meza*

RAZIEL F. ARCEGA

~ CONTRIBUTING WRITER ~

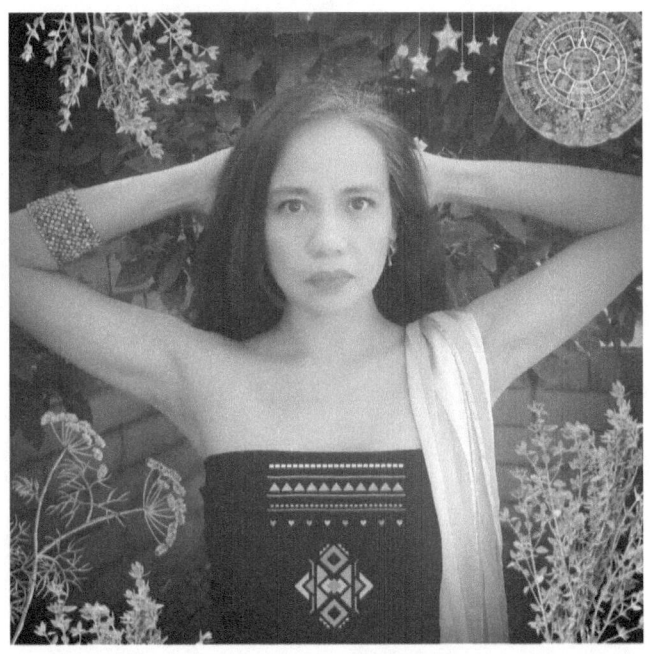

Raziel F. Arcega is a best-selling Co-Author on the collaborative book series Awakening Starseeds: Shattering Illusions Vol. 1, and a contributing writer for the forthcoming book, Infinite Cosmic Records: Sacred Doorways to Healing and Remembering with Maya The Shaman, and Pillars of Light: Stories of Goddess Activations™. (All books are created by Radhaa Publishing House.)

Raziel is a mother of two and a dynamic organizer within the Filipino-Asian community of Los Angeles, California. Her momprenuer business specializes in signage, banners, lighting, virtual event promo bags, client gifts, and drop shopping. Reach out to Raziel for your business needs, and she is here to serve you! For your promotional products, Business Events & Consulting email Raziel at: lnrpromotions@gmail.com

CHAPTER 10

LALITA GODDESS ACTIVATIONS™

Angelica

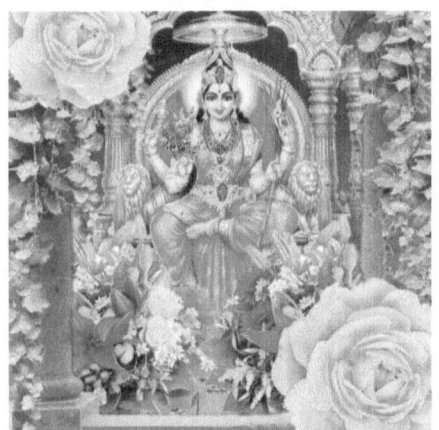

It's often hard to make sense of the pain this life brings, but that's what my Goddess Activations™ session with Radhaa gave me, a deeper understanding of. Along with peace, emotional cleansing, a deep meaning, and tremendous light. I have known Radhaa for more than a decade, followed her work, and read her Galactic Goddess book. We'd had deep conversations as dear friends.

I'd long known that Radhaa was wise, eons beyond her years, and a gifted seer, speaker, and writer, but I was amazed at the time of my healing session, the day of my Goddess Activations™ to discover what a gifted healer and clairvoyant she is.

The Epic Soulmate Connection

I'd just had to let go of my beloved partner because he had toxic behaviors in this life; it was soul-crushing to me. Even though we undoubtedly shared a deep connection and had some of the most intimate and tender moments imaginable, he was destructive to our sacred bond when triggered. Both he and I could see that he was sabotaging the relationship like some other force overtook him, and we had tried desperately to break the cycle, repeatedly and unsuccessfully. It was time to let go, but it felt like ripping apart every fiber of my being to do so.

I deeply understood all of his wounding and what he needed to do to heal because much of it had been similar to mine in earlier years, so I picked my sensitive self up from obliteration every time he destroyed us – injured and exhausted, I powered on because I knew and loved his soul. He was desperate to make it right. What Radhaa saw and shared in my session shed light on all of this.

The first time this man and I met, almost three years before the day of our final breakup, we both acknowledged that our eyes were familiar to each other on the first date! He interlaced his fingers in mine, stared into my eyes, and I felt a love that was ancient (even though at the time I wasn't sure I even believed in past lives.) When Radhaa revealed we were picking up where we left off in previous lives, I realized we'd always known this at some level, from day one. We fell deeply in love, both proclaiming, "we'd found each other." We both had never felt this before.

My beloved and I would sometimes meet in our dreams (we lived apart), which was confirmed the following day or often immediately, texting each other at three AM when we both woke up from this powerful rendezvous. "Did you feel/see that?" I'd text in the middle of the night. His reply would pop up immediately, and vice-versa: I'd wake up from experience and look, and he would have just texted "wow." In-person, we could feel each other's energy and sometimes even hear each other's thoughts. How do you break a bond like this? With the power of the Goddess!

Only a sliver of his soul was available to me in this life, and many times, darker parts overtook him, and he was hurtful to me. It seemed so simple to me. We belong together. How could he let anything stand in our way? But each time my love and devotion, and vulnerability were violated, the pain and my subsequent setting off boundaries brought us both to our knees, and we charted a healing path with intricate plans for protection and healing. But each time, unleashed destruction surfaces again before the healing could take place. I became so battle-worn when he faltered again, I knew I had to end it. He broke my trust and knew I could not go on.

The Insight with Goddess Lalita

Radhaa invited the Hindu Goddess, Lalita, into our session, who explained that what I'd thought of as my "soulmate man," though his core was divine and powerful, was addicted to the oppression and suffering this life had dealt him before we met. He had deep psychic wounds, but something inside of him would not let him heal, "face himself," and live the dream that we both envisioned, and as it turned out, we had lived before! Thanks to Radhaa's Goddess Activations™, I have complete peace with it all now because I understand this man and what we were to each other across time.

"He was asleep," the Goddess explained. Subsequently, at the mercy of the coping mechanisms, he used, in turn, to deal with the suffering and oppression he subjected himself to--a vicious, miserable cycle that the Goddess said I was enabling by standing by him. She said that the most loving thing I could do was release him so he would have a clear choice – face his "stuff" or continue sleeping, self-soothing, and self-destructing (but no longer at my expense). She gave me so much understanding and peace, realizing that I wasn't wrong to believe in him all this time and to see all the divine power in him, as well as to see what exactly he needed to heal. It was truly there. But I had to accept that he didn't fully believe in it and therefore couldn't sustain the strength to overcome his demons, addictions, and self-doubt. He didn't have confidence in his power and divinity. The contrast between what I saw in him and his behavior had been my undoing because it was so opposite to the man I knew in my soul from the past life we'd had together on the prairie.

The Cord Cutting Ritual

After the breakup and before Radhaa's Goddess Activations™, I did lots of meditation, Emotional Freedom Technique (EFT) "meridian tapping," and a classic "cutting the (energetic) chords," ritual, previously given to me by another gifted healer and seer, Gabriela Zigby, AKA "The Angel Witch." During the cord-cutting ritual, you invoke the archangels to help you remove each chord that binds you to each of the seven Chakra Centers between you and the person with whom you need to disconnect your energy. I'd become adept at this type of work and had powerful tools in my healing toolkit as a Master Practitioner of EFT.

I got to work on my battered psyche, but this time, the destruction might have gone too far; my healing abilities were compromised, and at the same time, despite his betrayal and dysfunction in this life, my bond with this man across time was epic. I was in over my head in terms of healing myself and felt powerless.

The cord-cutting ritual normally takes 20-30 minutes, but these chords between my man and me were more like tree trunks in the visualization. This time, the ritual took over two hours, and that was the second try.

During the first try, I confronted my inner child, who clung to him like the plush "blanky" that I was attached to as a child. This young girl refused to let go during the cord-cutting. "No! she screamed in desperation at me (my "executive self") and the angels. "HE IS MY HOME!"

My higher self gently but firmly said to her, "Do you want to die?" (because if we continued with him, this was the reality: soul death.) But she had no comprehension of such and refused to look at how he was currently showing up in this life. I was so drained from this struggle with her. I had to try the ritual again another night.

The second try, after two hours of working with Archangel Michael and Archangel Rafael, who wrapped their loving wings around that little girl, she finally accepted, letting her hand slip out of soulmate man's hand, and fell with grief into the wings of the angels, like being put on life support. They hold her still.

The Emotional Clearing

I was heartbroken, but I still felt my beloved in every cell of my body and fiber of my being, and I felt "in my DNA"! These words came to me long before my session with Radhaa, making perfect sense given what the Goddess revealed! With the angels' help, as well as the Goddess Kali, who I'd embraced previously, I cut all the chords from each Chakra, but not without the staggering pain that felt strangely like losing a child, and I would find out in Radhaa's session the reason for that. In the cutting the chords ritual, the divine Archangel Michael assists in pulling the chords that bind us out of my beloved and myself. As we tried to pull them out of him, he resisted so sadly and didn't fight. Still, the innocent little boy in him who only wanted to be connected to me gazed into my eyes with longing and confusion (even though, in reality, the man had appeared to discard me). "Don't do it," he pleaded during the ritual. "We don't have to do this."

But we did have to do it. The warrior Goddess Kali was in charge. I'd never have had the heart to pull the chords out of him, with his inner child pleading with me, gazing into my soul. But the Goddess Kali could! She was a force of sacred destruction.

The cutting of the chord was done, and this got to me. I knew it was killed or be killed (kill the attachment, or be psychically, spiritually, and possibly physically destroyed). It felt like killing my baby– I had to look away and ask Kali to do the dirty work. I could barely function, but I was a shell. There were gaping wounds where the tree-trunk chords had connected at each chakra center. I knew I needed Radhaa's healing modality.

Goddess Activations™ Session with Radhaa

As we started the Goddess Activations™ session, Radhaa explained that while my cord-cutting ritual had been successful, there were different layers of chords between me and my beloved. We have to dissolve them all across all time and space for me to let go fully. She saw that we had many lifetimes together, and then, as we were cutting the multiple layers of chords, she saw something astounding that explained so much about our bond and why detaching from him felt like killing my baby. There were umbilical cords between us! I had not shared with Radhaa previously those details about the inner child from my first chord cutting attempt, but when she said that I had been his mother and he had been mine in past lives, it all made sense. That's how the little girl part of me saw it. Of course, I realize we could call these "daddy issues" from childhood in this life, and that could certainly be a fair lens through which to see it. Still, it doesn't capture the complexity or the depth of this particular relationship, and I hadn't had "daddy issues" before this relationship or with anyone else.

This umbilical bond also helped me understand why his less-than-cherishing behaviors in our relationship cut me to the core. Likewise, for him, the pain he'd experienced with me cut him deeply and caused him to react in destructive ways to perceived threats of abandonment. Instead of immediately simply rejecting bad behavior and moving on like I normally would have in a romantic relationship, my soul was in shock and couldn't accept the reality of the violation. It was for him to treat me with anything other than cherishing, protecting, and the deepest love. I would react with fierce indignation, which only made him more afraid of being abandoned. It explained why there was so much profound love and so much trauma when our sacred connection was violated in this life. What otherwise might have been viewed by couples simply as "a fight" (though not a functional one) for us was a stunning violation of that part of our bond, that of a mother. It felt like such brutality should never enter into that relationship. We are to be the safe place to each other, "home," just as my inner child had decried during the chord cutting!

Radha helped me release it all. She began clearing, not just the chords but all the emotional stuff: "insecurity, pain, jealousy, grief, anger, sadness, despair, betrayal." Every word Radhaa uttered during this part of the session was spot on – targeting every emotional toxin in me that needed to be cleansed — maybe 100 emotions, and they came out in tears, and breath and even slight rocking at times, hands tightly clenched in prayer. They were so specific. When she said the word "horror," I broke down weeping (even more) as I had indeed felt horror the moments I had seen the betrayals he committed, though I hadn't placed that emotion exactly. Radhaa, through the Goddess, accurately saw far more in me than I even saw myself. She said, "Give Lalita your pain," and I did.

The Goddess Spoke

The Goddess Lalita spoke through Radhaa. She spoke to my heart's greatest needs to understand what seemed inexplicable, explaining that this man truly loved me. Ultimately, he could not believe in his power and was powerless to change, heal, and fully be himself. That felt true, but I asked how he could be so cruel at times, and she had much gentleness for him when she shared, "that's only when you were in the way of his addiction or when you were pushing him to look at things he wasn't ready to face. He always loved you." Instantly I saw an aggregate of every agonizing experience with him, and I knew it was true. I felt his love through it all. I knew Lalita was right, and it was deeply healing.

I finally understood and felt at peace with everything. Radhaa said it was important to know that I didn't fail. It hit me hard! It was visceral as I let go of that feeling of failure. The Goddess knew that I felt it was destiny to heal and thrive with this man for most of three years, but she gave me so much comfort in letting that go and knowing that I did everything I could, but it was his choice for not choosing us. I didn't have to make it work anymore, something I'd been burdened with for so long with so much conviction that I'd put myself in harm's way for that quest. I was free! I had clarity and was infused with so much wisdom and strength. I felt Lalita become a presence within me, enhancing my core self and bringing in the healing light.

The Homecoming

Then, Lalita showed Radhaa and me the past life I had with my Beloved. It washed away so much pain. We were a pioneer couple arriving at a pristine, lush prairie. As she described us, I began to see even more. I saw us struggling through treacherous travels to get there, and all the while, this man's essence was the same spirit, energy, and personality I'd fallen in love with within this life. He was divinely masculine indeed navigating, planning, taking charge, powering through, protecting me.

Depending on each other for survival, a bonded team mirrored how I felt about him in this life. In our prairie life, he was my hero every day, and I was his cherished angel. I saw us sitting together by fire as we celebrated our arrival. I looked into his soul through the same sparkling eyes he had on our first date in this life. We'd made it! In this prairie, we would thrive, and he, my champion, had led us here. These were the eyes I'd also felt were ancient and magical. The feeling in my heart was the same that I'd felt throughout our relationship: he was home.

This prairie vision fully illuminated why it was difficult to let go of him through the tumultuous human conflict and violations. I was trying to get us back to the prairie! A life in which we'd overcome all, together. That's why we had felt destined and why it was so brutal to let go. I'd thought we were meant to make it, and yet, in this life, he was destructive and not even fully available, leaving me in a difficult state! It explained why those eyes betraying me were in such trauma because they would never have. But Lalita gave me peace to disconnect from him and be open to other dreams in this life. It was finally okay to let go because we'd already had it! What I had thought of as losing, I got to relive with Lalita. I realized this destined guest had already been complete! I got to experience all the joy and profound love that we'd had in the past life through the Goddess's vision, which allowed me to save myself from what reality was a toxic relationship in this life. Lalita helped me stake my home within myself and let go of him.

The Aftermath

I felt my heart Chakra healing during the session with Radhaa and for days and weeks after. There is occasional pain to release when I remember something specific, but I call on the connection with the Goddess, and she helps me through it. Lalita's joyful and playful spirit shines through in my personality now. More doors are opening in various areas, and life is expanding in every way. I'm a more playful and relaxed mom, more creative and productive in my work, and I feel ready to find my sacred partner for this life. My heart is bigger because of its scars, and because I'm committed to protecting it, my heart is now safe. That safety made it possible through my healing journey begets openness, and openness makes everything possible. I'm most grateful to Radhaa for connecting me with Goddess Lalita. She is with me still, and I know the best is yet to come.

Saying:

"The repression of the feminine has led to a planet on the edge of collapse. The re-emergence is going to be a dance to behold."

~ Clare Dakin

ANGELICA

~ CONTRIBUTING WRITER ~

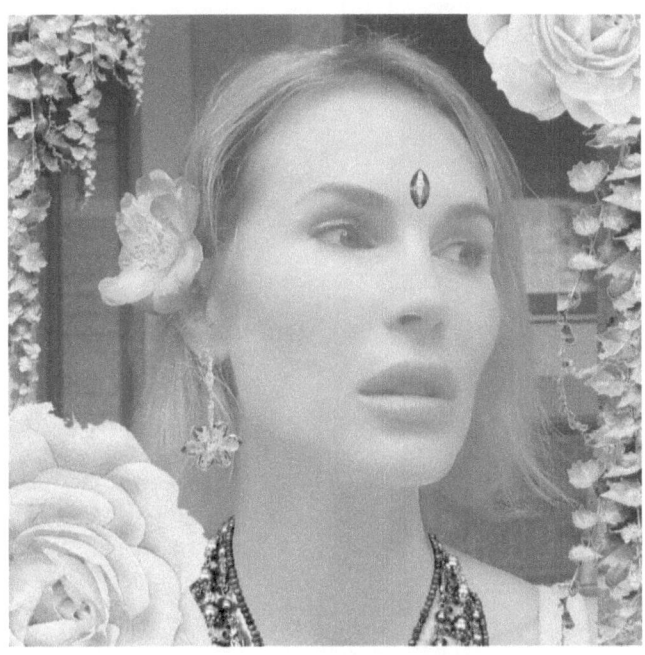

Angelica is a Journalist devoted to looking at parenting dilemmas through the lens of interdisciplinary science. Parenting Coach. Eternal Student. Mom of two little angels.

Saying:

"There's an entire spectrum of the Divine Feminine for us all to explore – and it truly is a personal journey of integration."

– Carly Stephan

CHAPTER 11

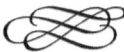

AKHILANDESHWARI GODDESS ACTIVATIONS™

Shakti Devi

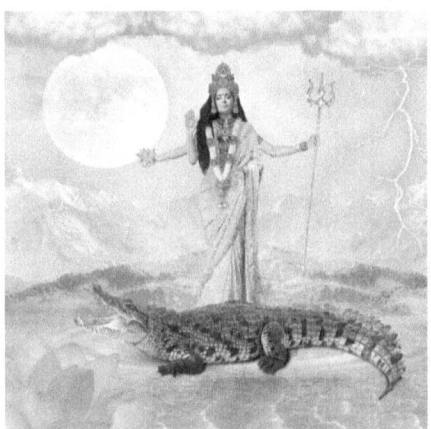

Namaskar, everyone, how beautiful it is to be alive and feel everything so deeply, even if it's exhausting yet fulfilling to our being. Thank you for existing and sharing the goodness of your heart with the world. Let me start with how grateful I am to be part of this wonderful soul revolution by stepping into our divinity and tapping into our inner Goddess, then embodying that gift that will bless others with healing and understanding.

Journey Within

It's been eight years since I woke up from a deep slumber. Okay, let me tell you a little glimpse of my spiritual journey where everything started. At a very young age, life has been hard, every day feels like torture both mentally and physically when you're being bullied, and yeah, it's exhausting! It feels like you're being cursed, and you constantly want to escape from that horror. The only way I've been thinking of is to end this life and end the nightmare. That's my mindset when I was young and naive, but I am grateful to move out of this mindset because there's a force stopping me from doing so. Later on, as I matured, I realized that when you finally get tired of something, don't just quit; instead, let the divine intervention lead the way. It can be a very long journey. Hence, it's important to have faith so strong that you can move mountains and ask the Universe for the strength to walk away from trivial-mundane realities that hurt the soul and have clear guidance as one continue unraveling the path we're heading to.

It's been a wonderful journey from the past few years of knowing and connecting with a dear friend and mentor, Ate Radhaa. *"In the Philippines, where I came from, it's a tradition to call a caring guide, Ate, or Auntie, a sign of honor and respect."* Ate Radhaa supported me and reminded me that nothing was wrong with me or that I was not weird and everything was uniquely normal. She has this motherly energy, such caring, loving, and very supportive nature. Reflecting on the past, I can say I'm very proud of the process and progress I've been making, and I am beyond thankful for all the beautiful souls I met and connected with.

So there you go, fast forward to the session. I was sitting in my half lotus meditative state, excited and curious about what Goddess Activations™ will bring.

Goddess Activations™ Session

I started the session. Upon hearing Ate Radhaa's sweet soothing voice, I felt her magical vibrations as always. She asked me to have three deep breaths. Suddenly I felt an abrupt increase of energy around me. It felt warm. My body began to feel tingly. The sensation is crawling at the bottom of my feet, going upward to the top of my head. It's like something is being activated until Ate Radhaa told me it was the light codes being poured into my physique when she started to call upon my Goddess Akhilandeshwari, oh Goddess! It felt surreal. My body felt numb, cold, and warm altogether. My heart center started to vibrate as if someone was squeezing it. It made me want to cry, but after a moment, without even noticing, my tears started to stream down my face.

I can sense that there's a lot of things going on inside of me. There's pressure on the top of my head. Ate Radhaa explained that there's a lot of purification taking place in my being: heart, mind, and soul. My soul fragments are being recalibrated. She cleared energy cords that are no longer serving my highest potential. After the clearing and pulling off the unwanted energy cords, I felt so light, like all the burden accumulated from the past incarnations were suddenly lifted off. Ate Radhaa is indeed a very powerful healer and a carrier of the Goddess Codes™. Every word she spoke brought me goosebumps, and I know it's real and came from the Divine.

Even a crazy thing happened. This physical mind is trying to be logical about what's happening. It's like ego thoughts keep on popping out, but dah? Who cares, everything is so amazing, and even though it's beyond explanation somehow deep within me, in my soul, it's clearly understood. It was Divine! I am exactly where I need to be. The experience itself was incredibly remarkable, a once-in-a-lifetime opportunity.

Soul Imprint

Ate Radhaa speaks directly to my soul. She is bold and humorous at the same time. She brings clarity and light into my being. The entire session cracked me open, and it made me experience what it is like to unleash my inner Goddess and step into my divinity. She emphasizes that I have to be fully aware of my power, because I've been suppressed and must acknowledge it. The reason why is because I've been bullied and betrayed by the people that I loved, yet, it doesn't stop me from being more gentle, understanding, and learning what unconditional love means.

I truly believe that's why and how I was able to connect to Ate Radhaa.

Every message that Ate Radhaa has spoken has made me realize more about what I wanted to be in this life, how I wanted to spend my lifetime, and my purpose. It makes total sense why I wanted to be in service to others, be a storyteller, and be a helping hand to my fellow women and men.

The Activation: Goddess Akhilandeshwari & Falling in Love with the Broken, not Broken Goddess

I chose to experience the Goddess Activations™ because I wanted to learn more about myself. I am curious about what it brings. I knew I was ready to unlock what's within me to experience this shift and be fully rooted in it because the guide finally appeared! Ate Radhaa was the perfect healer for me to have this session to align me with the right Goddess I needed to connect with. I am so grateful I happened to experience this kind of session and being divinely connected at the right time.

The moment Ate Radhaa introduced Goddess Akhilandeshwari, *"the broken and not broken Goddess,"* I fell in love with this Goddess because I definitely can identify and connect with her in my journey. The brokenness that I experienced guided me and led me into this path that I am walking right now.

Goddess Akhilandeshwari works tremendously with my heart chakra. She opens it up a little more and makes it much stronger but also gentler, and my solar plexus activates it a little more so that I can fully step into my power. By the time Ate Radhaa told me that Akhilandeshwari was so grateful to assist me and have this connection, she would be glad to work beside me, and "*I am worthy of receiving and activating all the gifts that will help me assist others in their healing.*" It brought me to tears, and it felt like *"someone was hugging me but in spirit."*

The whole session was incredible. I let everything flow; it's overwhelming with the surge of energy so strong that it makes my body feel tingling up to the point it was numb, or perhaps I feel weightless. It makes me feel emotions that I can't even name. It makes me realize more how worthy I am of love, care, bliss, and accepting the feeling of being broken with an open heart, embracing my shadows with gladness fully because they are one of the most important ingredients that balance and color my life.

Sacred Journey

We're almost halfway to the end of our session. I continue to feel like floating into thin air while my eyes are closed, but I can see with my mind's eye a vibrant color of blue, sparkling golds, and I even smell a fragrance so familiar, yet I can't put a name on it, but I can imagine it's feeling of sweetness. Images were starting to show up, symbols and patterns of colors that made me feel emotional. I used to have these feelings of supernatural phenomena, but I can say that this is much different and more exciting than those experiences. The activation is very welcoming, and I feel tranquility vibrate all around me. The energies surrounding me are amazing, I can feel something in the realm of possibility, and the unknown opens widely. The multidimensional me is fully switched on, and yeah! That was beyond! Everything presented to me is what I need, and this is a clear message that never doubt the Divine.

Everything is being written in the book of life, even before we choose to land here on Earth. There is no such thing as coincidence. I believe that when it's time for us to walk and serve our purpose, we can open ourselves up and be brave to face whatever is in front of us.

It is because turning away or escaping it and it will never be doing us any good.

If you think that the Universe is punishing you, let me be the light. This is a living proof I am able to share my realizations.

"The Universe is so kind, even though you may feel you've been put in troubles, maybe it appears like that, and you are being punished, but only if you know how beautiful it is to appreciate its lessons. It's like a head-start and power-ups later when you finally realized it and spent your life being a light that will show others how they can find their strength, courage, healing and light."

Imagine making a ripple effect, an echo not only to the people you've made contact with but to the whole Universe. And finally, making heaven on Earth, where we seek healing and use our downfall, our brokenness as a form of strength to get up and find wholeness again, help support others rather than passing this brokenness to pollute others. This vision with Goddess Akilandeswari has given me so much inspiration to move on in my life and look at the bright side of it. It is a gift for me to get to know Goddess Akilandeswari through Ate Radhaa!

Ate Radhaa continued to say, *"Today as we move forward and there's a lot of shifting and recalibration happening because we're at the point of mass awakening, lots of dark/heavy stagnant energy is finally being released after a long period of captivity and being freed as our fellow souls are stepping out and seeking for the new light and realizing their true essence."*

I remember when I told Ate Radhaa, I saw a blue light. She laughed and immediately said that Archangel Michael was there guiding and protecting me. That's the divine masculine being present. She said that I got plenty of spirit guides, ascended masters, galactic family, and ancestors that wanted to be known for their presence. They wanted me to know that I am guided and supported in this magical journey.

> "In experiencing my sacred journey with a Goddess through Ate Radhaa, it is important to share our stories and make this kind of healing known, to spread the Goddess Activations™ to the world because it creates a total change that brings guidance and self-knowing."

Important Message

> "The session is beyond expectation; Ate Radhaa is truly exceptional."

It is such a great honor to be part of this league, a warrior of love, holder of the pillar of light. For some, it might sound unreal, and it makes no sense, and others may even want to block it to stop this message. Still, knowing this brings hope, motivation, security, and peace within makes me believe more in the unknown. It gives me all the possibilities to think of and allows me to take full responsibility for my actions. But then, always keep in mind that you're free to believe as you desire and do whatever you want to choose.

My father died eight years ago, and he played a major role in my spiritual awakening. Ate Radhaa made our session so special because she also conveyed a wonderful message from my father that he wanted me to know that he appreciates everything I've done, and he's proud of what person I've become. That made the session more special and memorable that I will treasure this forever.

"MOSAIC"
By: Shakti Devi

I call upon all the scattered and molded pieces of myself
Left with kisses and bruises
With the taste so bitter and the taste of the sweetest nectar that gives bliss
I honor everything that these hands gave birth
I am enough.
The water of life into these powerful palms
With every touch, healing resides.
I am worthy.
I carry the seed of life.

I carry the codes of light.
Into the mother's womb, I take rest.
I am fierce.
The fire that covers me, my passion ignites.
The grass that grows all over me, I've found my home.
I am free.
The wind that carries the message, I sing and listen.
She taught me to be calm instead of putting up resistance.
I am beautiful.
I am sensual.
Upon dwelling in the darkness, a new light arises.
I am glorious.
I am in control
When I thought I was just a broken glass, a scattered piece
She reminded me that I am a work of art indeed,
I am a masterpiece.

I can't thank Ate Radhaa enough for letting me experience her Goddess Activations™ and for being my mentor. It allows me to open myself to a deeper aspect of sovereignty and self-knowledge. Namaskar.

SHAKTI DEVI

~ CONTRIBUTING WRITER ~

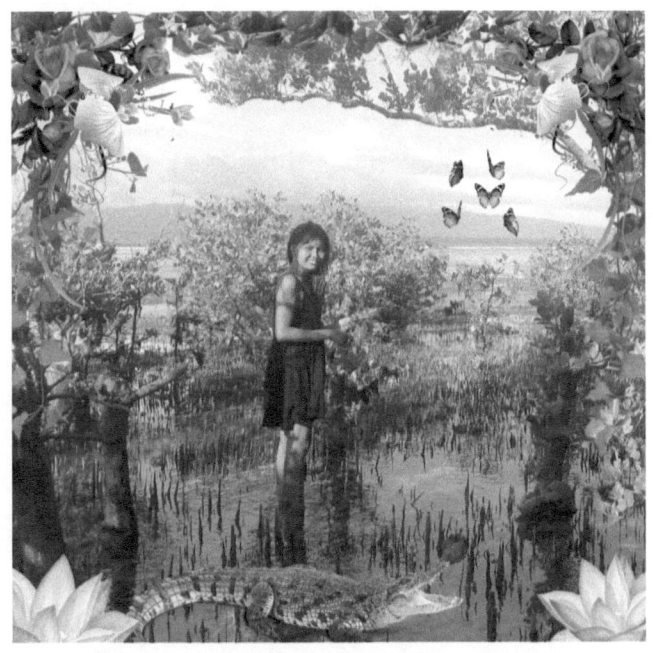

Shakti Devi is from Maharlika, known as the Philippines. She is a Massage Therapist, A Tantric Meditator, A Hand-crafter, an Artist, A student, and a teacher of life. As a seeker of her own deepest truth, she is also a lover of all things animate and inanimate. Shakti Devi is a Believer in Universalism. She loves to read and expand her mind. Observer of its Consciousness, or let say, "A soul that keeps on enjoying and exploring its roller coaster and bike ride-like-life experiences.

Shakti Devi radiate unconditional love for every being while she's still here with "Mother Gaia's Creation." A star-soul incarnated as a woman.

CHAPTER 12

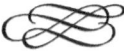

ABUNDANTIA GODDESS ACTIVATIONS™

Brenda Lainof

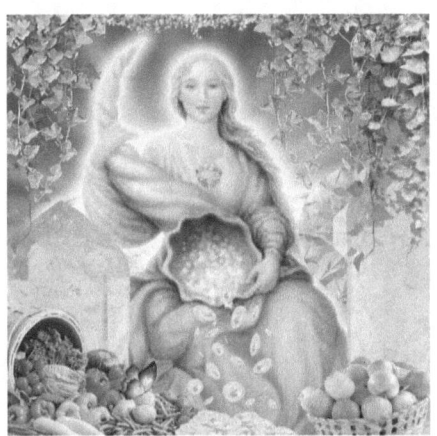

I have been affected by energies that have tarnished and shut down my soul for many lifetimes, and it has affected me physically and at a soul level. Little did I realize how vital it was to have the Goddess activations™, Abundantia, for abundance.

Abundantia, also called Abundita, was **a divine personification of abundance and prosperity in ancient Roman religion.** The name

Abundantia means plenty or riches, and this name is fitting as Abundantia was a goddess of abundance, money flow, prosperity, fortune, valuables, and success. She would help protect your savings and investments.

Friendship with Radhaa

I have had the opportunity to exchange our stories, life experiences with Radhaa, as a co-author in "Awakening Starseeds, Stories Beyond the Stargate, Vol. 2. I was thrilled to receive a transmission from Radhaa. I did not know what to expect! And how fitting it was to Abundantia.

After the transmission, I was confident that I was on the right path and that I have an important message to share with the world, for ALL of the Light Workers of the World who are struggling with their abundance, who have signed up to be on earth at this exact moment, to assist humanity.

Background

As a very young girl, as far back as around the age of five, I realized that I was "different" and had always felt "different" from my biological siblings. Looking back in time, I did not fit in with my earthly family. *I felt like a misfit, and this misfit feeling carried throughout all of my lifetimes.*

You see, it was very ingrained in my father's upbringing that we were to portray a certain image of being affluent. I remember hearing comments throughout the years about how my father was referred to as "money bags." And these comments felt like daggers and darts, perhaps out of jealousy, insecurity from neighbors, friends, some family members?

In my young mind, I questioned why would anyone refer to my father as "money bags?" What does that mean? I never considered our family wealthy, not at all! And found the reference somewhat offensive and truly puzzling. And yet, there was undoubtedly a certain persona that our family exuded, portrayed, within the community that we were "financially affluent." A status that I certainly could not identify with. As an intuitive young girl, it just felt "wrong," "dirty," "fake."

Yes, we lived in a lovely home, certainly did not lack for anything materially, but I never regarded my family as "wealthy." I do remember feeling somewhat uncomfortable, a sense of awkwardness, this false perception of being affluent.

"I now realize that I have always rejected an abundance of money...."

Many years later, after a challenging first marriage, single parent, I remarried for the 2nd time. My husband worked in the Corporate World, living in what I regarded as a financially abundant state. We both had great paying jobs, work opportunities in international countries, a beautiful primary home, and a vacation home in a stunning desirable location too. We are also able to provide all of the material needs for our blended family.

On the outside world, everything looked great! We had it all. However, inside my mind, I was struggling to keep it all together. I felt like a fraud, just as I did as a young child. I found myself in a state of being stressed out, working long hours, spreading myself too thin, personal relationship suffering, and my health on a SLOW, STEADY decline for many years.

Transmission

In my transmission with Radhaa, she intuited that I had made an oath as a young girl. This oath was that I would never be looked upon with evil eyes, envious eyes like my father did, and feel bad, dirty, shamed. Radhaa revealed in my transmissions that I had many incarnations, many lifetimes where a particular program had been installed through a holographic package.

"Dark energies hijacked me!"

It was like an inversion where the dark receives energy, and the light feels deficient. I am and have been the "light."

"And I have always been an empath!"

An empath is highly aware of those around them, to the point of feeling those emotions themselves. We see the world differently than other people, and we take on their emotions unknowingly at some level!

But it's not just emotions. As empaths, we can feel physical pain and often sense someone's intentions or where they're coming from. In other words, empaths seem to pick up on many of the lived experiences of those around them.

Goddess Abundantia

Abundantia poured gold liquid light over my crown chakra, down through my mind. In the process, it melted away all artificial programs that I was ready to release ~ *felt energy gently pouring throughout my entire "being."* Energy continued, pushing and pulling up false beliefs and thoughts.

"I AM ready to INSTALL New Belief that I DESERVE to be a financially abundant Light Worker."

Clearing and Installing

Throughout the entire process of installing, "I AM abundant," Radhaa heard the words "ancestral, war, struggle" and asked for those memories, all of the inherited emotions, to dissolve, clear, and release. Thoughts showing up: "I AM not good enough, and I AM not worthy. It's too hard to be abundant, and I have to work hard to make it happen. That struggle is all there is." Abundantia removed beliefs from my body and reprogrammed my DNA and RNA.

The Goddess Activations™ downloads came through. "I AM good

enough. Worthy and deserving. Easy to be abundant. Easy to be in an abundant flow. Know how to be in an abundant flow. Possible to be in abundant flow and throughout my DNA and RNA. Downloading a feeling of grace and ease to every cell of my body down to toes, fingertips, crown chakra, back, and front."

In the session I discovered my past lives. I had made vows of poverty as a Monk in Tibet, a nun in Europe (a lot of tingling in my head), had many lifetimes, and as an evolved soul, returned to earth and volunteered over and over again. There was always a theme of devotion to the Source, Creator, God. The sad disclosed part is that I had disowned abundance as my birthright.

Radhaa affirmed: "*I am here to rebalance the truth and recode I AM abundant.*"

Abundantia through Radhaa as a conduit folded in my timelines, sprinkled my timelines with gold, revoked all contracts, and marked them as completed in the Akashic records. All of the vows that I had declared no longer served me and installed "safe to let them go" calibrated cellular memory from all of these lifetimes.

Such a flow of energy, as Abundantia cleared beliefs that "money excludes people," "money ruins relationships," "money may hurt people just as I witnessed in my childhood."

Transmission continued: That Angelic aspect wanted to support me, "I AM an Earth Angel," to make these waves as I never truly valued the impact I have had over hundreds of clients throughout the past 20 years. Showing that I am here as a way-shower, but I also deserve to enjoy abundance! Lead the way, break the patterns!

"Activating abundance code in my being and will be transmitting this energy that it's Safe to be Abundant for Light Workers."

Abundantia continued to clear out beliefs and "feelings of being cheated," such as: "what's the point of having these gifts if I am not truly abundant?" Despair, bitterness, over-giving, not receiving, "this is as good as it gets?" Radhaa moved the energies throughout all past, present, future, parallel lifetimes, lineage, inherited, all heaviness lifted from lineage and sent back to the source to take care of it.

"I took in a few deep breaths and started to feel lighter, more optimistic."

The releasing continued, the disappointment of being "let down," the anger of pissed off, further burning out old programs in the root chakra and transmuting all of the stuck stagnant energy in chakras.

"The feeling of hopelessness started to dissipate."

It was replaced with anticipation, knowing that my journey as a Starseed is to heal further and clear all feminine programming that "women can't stand in their power" and transmute to "women can reclaim what they want, what they deserve!"

Truly grateful for the experience of Abundantia Goddess Activations™ and deep understanding. The transmission came through Radhaa and Abundanita. Until our time together, I never realized why I was so stuck on creating fuller abundance. And so GRATEFUL for her guidance and clearings! I, too, look forward to bringing people to a place of acceptance, joy, and grace as to their power of abundance.

Realization

Through the deep dive with Radhaa, I now realize that living financial abundance not only deepens my personal life and how this gift of abundance is truly every living soul's birthright. I suggest that is only one part of life's puzzle.

"It is Safe to be Abundant as a Light Workers"

Mystery Unfolding

Appreciating What I Have
Is one way to turn a Rock Into Gold
My Suffering into Meaningful Aspect
Of Mystery Unfolding
To Come My Way
Transforms How Life
Continually Flows as Abundance

Saying:

"The deep Feminine, the mystery of consciousness, She who is life, is longing for our transformation as much as we are. She holds back, allowing us free reign to choose, nudging us occasionally with synchronicities, illness, births, and deaths… But when we make space for Her, she rushes into all the gaps, engulfing us with her desire for life and expression. This is what She longs for, this is what we are for: experiencing the Feminine through ourselves. We simply need to slow down and find where to put our conscious attention. And it is this, this willingness to look again, this willingness to put consciousness into our places of unconsciousness, to express what we have always avoided, which starts the process of unblocking, so that She may flow through."

– **Lucy H. Pearce**

BRENDA LAINOF

~ CONTRIBUTING WRITER ~

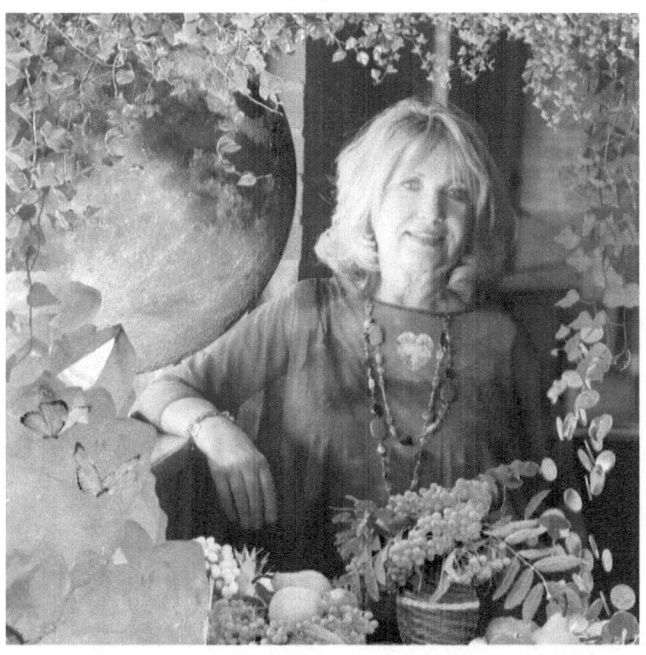

Brenda Lainof is an intuitive guide and assists in clearing negative emotions and chronic health conditions, emotional and mental self-sabotage. Once she intuits what creates unease in your body, Brenda energetically works with you to dissolve that unease, dis-ease, and low-frequency vibration. She works with numerous modalities and uses the most appropriate modality that is needed at the moment. Every client is different, and she taps into you as to what you are READY FOR!

Brenda help identify accurately and assist the body to self-heal with the appropriate modality and download applicable Light Language. www.brendalainof.com

CHAPTER 13

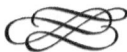

FREYA GODDESS ACTIVATIONS™

Y'Shell Esta

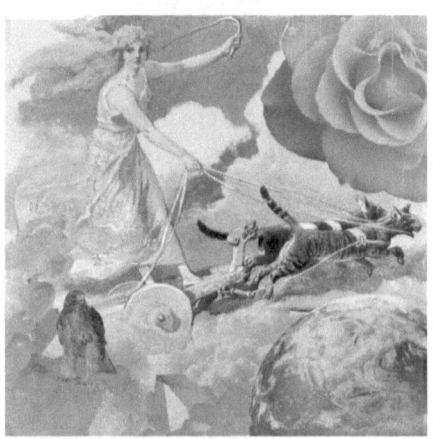

Triumphant Healer Activated

It has been three years since I have been pushed outside of my comfort zone, spiritually. This zone was a co-dependent relationship of repressive and reactive natures, a decade of being in my own personal Spanish 'novella' ending in divorce. I remember over those years the disrespect, self-expression issues, lack of trust, inability to speak my feelings, repressed feelings, giving my power to another person, his anger and rage, a lot of walking on eggshells, and carrying these heavy loads of trauma. I became a shadow version of myself, broken in my inner self.

Did I need to see a therapist? It was insisted, "I was blamed" for my insecurities. But what about him? I started to question myself about everything. Which then had him replying that I didn't trust him. Did I begin not to believe him or not trust him? I questioned my actions a lot. I learned to tuck my feelings away and have better control over them. I tried to prevent a situation I didn't want to be in, an experience where it ended up in a fight, a fight that may have led to rage. This rage led to him putting me down, only later to tell me not to take it personally. I was not too fond of the energy that lingered after our fights. It felt like I was playing a game I had no chance of winning. I didn't even know I was "playing" until it was too late. I was accused of being crazy or abusive for reacting to his abuse, thus playing the 'victim role.'

This relationship evolved cyclically. As much as I insisted on staying together, hoping the next chapter would be different, it was worse than the one before. My dependency was the chronic neglect to gain approval, love, validation, and self-identity. Trauma bonding was real, too, in that past timeline. The trauma left my nervous system in complete dysregulation leading to dis-ease in my body. Looking back, I was constantly in a fight or flight trauma response in survival mode, not listening to my body that was screaming out to me. I had to take my spiritual healing seriously and stop all of it!

My friends and family wondered what happened to the woman who used to be so strong and energetic. I had frantically excused this behavior and could not acknowledge the painful truth behind my relationship, and something had changed. I'd spend hours on the phone, hoping for his afternoon text message or promised phone call, and I wouldn't make plans for the day to make sure I was available to him. It wasn't until after being separated and getting the support of my friends and family that I could begin to see everything more clearly.

Therapy taught me that I am not a product of my past or those circumstances but a product of my decisions today. Hence, the power to own my vulnerabilities, embrace them and carry them in the world as great gifts of beauty, love, and healing. Today, I am in a much happier space, leading a life filled with more meaning, joy, and connection. Knowing that I am the creator of my reality, I celebrate myself with freedom of expression. The most important relationship I have is with myself, shaping every relationship I have. My healing path is to remember, re-learn, and reconnect with myself, whereas before, I was conditioned to believe others created my sense of self. I continue to build healthier, authentic relationships with others. As I attune within myself more, I heal and let go of any co-dependent tendencies and move towards genuine, heart-centered relationships. Practice makes perfect.

It is a privilege to learn and love all my relations from this. The single greatest challenge in my life leading to my conscious evolution, written in my genetic profile, is Gene Key 4. Transcending my suffering moves from the shadow of intolerance to the highest essence of forgiveness; and, it is through the path of understanding. It is in direct partnership with my life's work, Gene Key 49, creatively expressing my full freedom to be myself without compromise moves from the shadow of reaction to the absolute zenith of my genetic potential of rebirth; and, it is the way I can achieve true recognition in life by revolution. It is a grand synthesis of practical wisdom to help guide us to a deeper understanding of ourselves and our true potential by the contemplation of Gene Keys (Rudd, 2015).

I was blind to the toxicity our relationship had become. It wasn't my job to detox toxic people, and it was my responsibility to detox the part of myself that resonated with their toxicity. We had an opportunity to grow together, and, unfortunately, what unfolded was the shadow side to this shadow behavior.

Kin 16 Yellow Electric Warrior Affirmation:
"I Activate in Order to Question
Bonding Fearlessness
I seal the Output of Intelligence
With the Electric tone of Service
I am guided by the power of Universal Fire."
– Dr. José Argüelles, PhD

Accelerated Radical Acceptance

Even now, sharing my interpretation of my experiences is me openly coming out of "my shell," an initiation of sorts. So not only is this an invitation from Radhaa for the Goddess Activations™ of Freya, but it's also an initiation from the Universe that I am invited into right now to embody fully and stand in my truth for leveling up. Freya is the perfect archetype that matches my personality for me to draw from. I can see reflections given her qualities, fierceness as a warrior and fullness as a nurturer. She is loving, kind, strong, and brave. She is an archetype from which I draw strength and perspective. Her qualities help her get through things no matter how afraid or heartbroken.

Freya, her name meaning Lady, is one of the preeminent deities in Norse mythology. She is the Earth Goddess of celebration, love, beauty, fertility, prosperity, war, and a Goddess of life and death. She rides in her chariot pulled by two mighty cats across the rainbow bridge connecting heaven and Earth. I let the peace of Freya enter my mind. She is here to remind me that the acceptance of defeat is not the end. She offers the gift of acceptance, knowing that there is nothing to resist right now. I accept. I can see with greater clarity and discernment, not taking this world so personally, that I do not have to fight at all. I surrender to what is and move to higher grounds from standing in the middle of all the chaos that once was.

Freya is also known as the archetypal völva (female Shaman), a practitioner of the magical arts of divination. She introduced the Gods to seidr, a form of art and ritual that could see events before they happened and allowed practitioners to change the future (McCoy,

2019). Since I know all the natures and characteristics of astrology, galactic signatures, and Gene Keys, I have the opportunity to access and activate elements of it that I need to do "to propel me to where I need to be" during these transformational days.

Showing me how to manifest my dreams, no matter how out of reach they may seem, remembering I am a powerful creative force. I am encouraged to embrace my Divine Feminine; feel my natural sensuality from the inside radiating out, delving into the very depths of my soul. When I am hard on myself for not living up to unrealistic standards set upon by my ego, I overlook the powerful and passionate Divine being that lives within every one of us. It is time I am bold and let my light shine, permitting myself to be authentically me.

As I step into my power, I am beautiful in confidence and grace. Freya is encouraging me to step into my gift of graciousness as a woman, a quality that every woman naturally possesses. I am a gracious person. Now I get to apply it across the board, especially with those particular relationships where there may still be conflict, thus giving me a chance to transmute it. And calling all my triggers "grace growers." If and when they present themselves, I ask myself how they can show me how to grow in grace, learning new ways to perceive in time and better to remain in peace than knowing why. A wise man and beloved friend told me that to be gracious; One must always say thank you. Always. Whether I agree or not, because it will immediately neutralize the intention.

I am compelled to model graciousness for my son in my role as his mother. My four-year-old sees how his mother and father choose to navigate real life, informing him how to communicate, make decisions, and take action. As a mother, I possess certain wisdom for his well-being to remain balanced.

"When we are very young, we learn how to feel about ourselves and life by the reactions of the adults around us" (Hay, 1999). From now on, my son needs and wants healthy parents who can show him what self-love is and instill in him a sense of self. He can understand that people behave towards him differently because of their own experiences and have nothing to do with him. I tell my son every day that I love him and am proud of him simply for being his true self. I talk with my son about all the positive aspects that make him unique. It is no wonder we teach our children manners and be polite at the ages three and four, so they begin to learn proper behavior while relating with others. After all, being polite means to unlock and radiate within our "potential light."

Even if his father comes off aggressively calling me names or sending me inappropriate text messages, I know now this is where grace can transcend because he isn't talking about me. Whoever he is identifying as me is a misidentification. He knows only of a particular interpretation of an experience he remembers and recalls of me. This interpretation doesn't mean that it is who I am right now. Here you see an example of one of many timelines playing out in the hologram that I have created, living out simultaneously with others. However, I have the choice to not engage in that and remain in my light, remaining gracious. It's not easy, but I have to transcend the nonsense. I am authentically, lovingly, gracefully approaching it this way because I ultimately want what's best for my son.

All I can do is keep the possibility open that my son's father will create a reality that aligns with mine. From a resonance standpoint, my choosing to approach it from grace will lift him by virtue into a space that I am creating. And it doesn't matter if he fights it or goes with it. My concern is what frequency I keep. Not letting anyone get the pleasure of pulling me out of my light. In the end, I am responsible for that.

I declared and decided to stop fighting my reality, stop responding with impulsive or destructive behaviors when things weren't going the way I wanted them to. And finally, I let go of the bitterness that may have kept me trapped in a cycle of suffering. This step forward was the beginning of my radical acceptance.

"Every intentional act is a magical act. Even the smallest action has a spin-off effect that travels out into the Universe. Actions made out of resentment or fear reinforce the Shadow frequency both in the world and in the individual. Indifferent acts reinforce indifference, whereas acts done in joy or Service create more joy." – *Richard Rudd*.

Unlocking My Higher Purpose

I was lucky to be a winner for a one-hour Goddess Code session in April 2017. I had the pleasure of meeting Radhaa 11 years ago and have seen her transform in her healing journey over the years. We finally dug up the root of my ancestral and childhood pain instantly during my first session, doing an energetic divorce with relationships.

It felt good knowing this was releasing and clearing out old patterns, ancient contracts my soul made that no longer align with who I came here to be, and emotional traumas in my luminous field. An energetic divorce is a spiritual tool and modality formulated to disentangle energetic ties and unhealthy attachments from the relationships, addictions, and life experiences that no longer serve us.

Precisely four years later, I was ready to activate a new Goddess, Goddess Freya. From this initial session with Radhaa, I heard the call before and witnessed all the beautiful synchronicities leading up to the activation. I knew I was ready to spiral up. To be a holder of light energy as a Pillar of Light for Los Angeles needs a lot of healing.

Radhaa has a magical divine Goddess approach, and at the same time, she is logical and genuine at explaining what is going on in your soul. I found her a truly gifted being who is kind and honest and made me feel safe, warm, and welcome in her presence. I was excited about our session, and it felt great to be connecting intimately again. We both acknowledge that I have done this before, and I already know pure love and paradise. And yet here I am again. This journey was never promised to be easy, but I must remember who I am: Divine Grace, even if it does not feel like that at times.

Setting my intentions, I ask the Universe, as I am tuning into my challenges, seen or unseen, here in the now, past, future, and parallel timelines, to please bring clear communication, clarity, and openness divine guidance. I ask for the courage to step out into becoming who I am meant to be here without any restrictions, conditionings, fear, or judgment. And, I welcome the activation of more mettā, more love, more gratitude, fun, celebration, and patience.

We began to ground and connect deep within the Earth, anchoring in my cords to the crystalline center, with my first opportunity to release and unload any baggage weighing me down and regenerating that healing life force back into me.

Activating my third eye, we head up into the cosmic light entering the bright light of the Universe and feeling safe to release again, moving through, shedding a layer of fear and judgment that I do not consent to anymore. Emerging from this luminous light, I feel the release and rebirth of energy. We continue traveling upward into the darkness, feeling complete freedom, joy, grace, ease, and expansion. As I look above, I see a beautiful luminous vast light moving closer into the heart of the divine creator Goddess. We pop into this space. I relax and feel the softness, safeness, and sacred space. We work at a higher level to not get interference. Also, it is protected and Activating here right down with me later into my physical body.

Radhaa continues calling on Goddess Freya to come forth. "We thank you for coming forward now." I take a deep breath then state my name three times, "Y'Shell Esta," each time, relaxing into this space to receive more. Goddess Freya is grateful that I have chosen her as she has chosen me. We have worked together in past lives and other incarnations. And she wants to get straight to it. "There are some lifetimes that you're ready to clear now. Lifetimes of persecution from misunderstandings. You are a beautiful divine feminine that has been hurt or shamed in some way that may be affecting your visibility at this time."

Radhaa brings forward the first timeline that is ready to clear, one that is all too familiar. There are beautiful aspects to it; "this feels like Ireland or lush green lands, an old castle of royalty;" I am the king and queen's daughter. Radhaa starts clearing. She tells me that I am a beautiful young woman. There is a theme of heartache and heartbreak because I fell in love with someone I was not supposed to. It's about this love and passion taken away for not being royalty. It isn't happening in my life right now, but there are echoes. Echoes, ghosts, shadows of grief, frozen tears, feelings that emotionally choked and held back parts of me because my truth wasn't honored, validated, and publicly destroyed. Radhaa clears out the hidden interferences from my soul mission in my heart to be more in my purpose, speak my truth, be in my voice and stand in my heart. I no longer consent to the reverberating past interference and echoes, affecting my ability to show how I am entirely meant to. This timeline resonated with me so much; I could feel the recurring cycles playing out again from the previous relationships I've shared in this life. A feeling of being silenced and my voice not being supported. Because I have done many healing sessions within the past few years with several teachers, detached from those experiences, I know they were lessons and opportunities to grow and learn.

Radhaa/Freya acknowledge that my vibration is so high and that I have done a great job to clear out these echoes and reverberation, but they are echoes, and the clearing needs to be consistent. Through Radhaa, Freya lined up all the many timelines with the same theme of heartbreak and silenced and distorted/leeched energy (energy vampires) that did not belong to me for us to witness—completely collapsing them all, so they don't ripple at the moment as we exist in the past, present, future, and parallel timelines all at once. Radhaa says: "Release, release, release, release." Marking that lesson as complete in my akashic records so I don't have to do it again! "Complete, complete, complete, complete."

Visuals flooded in on timelines completed. Radhaa moved in warrior momentum, Freya prepared for the next ancient clearing to dissolve. Black magic and curses. Breathing in Source light codes and breathing out, visually releasing these ancient reverberations through the breath. A Sanskrit mantra was given to me by Radhaa during this time for protection from the jealousy of others.

As Radhaa continued her sacred work, invisible black goo was removed from my auric field. I started to feel a tugging or rooted sensation in the right shoulder and right abdomen side. Radhaa shared that Freya brings this happy, laughing, smiley face Buddha and I imagine them coming into my shoulder. Thousands of roses start to bloom out of my right shoulder, blooming out the roots of any distortions. It is explained that the distorted energy is not mine. My previous partner's traumas formed the stress and burden I have been carrying. It is beautiful to let it go now. Freya brings in another happy, laughing, smiley face Buddha right into the shoulder with another thousand roses cleaning it up. It's just purging out emotional energy. One more time, as Radhaa suggested, but this time, getting both shoulders, my neck, and my head bringing in thousand blooming roses to clear my crown chakra, my throat chakra, and both of my shoulders. Guan Yin of Divine Compassion appears, bringing the Lotus flower into my crown chakra blooming open.

Radhaa assured me that my job is to keep rising, exactly what I have been doing, and hearing the message that I am completely on track, anchoring in my work. Building up with a lot of momentum behind me to continue my journey and upcoming projects. Radhaa can see the rainbow spectrum of light connecting from heaven and Earth. I am on "the ground crew," and this rainbow light is coming down through me and then out of me like a crystal. I shared with her that I have been doing a meditation to generate the Circumpolar Rainbow Bridge of Universal World Peace, holding this pillar of light in these dark and dense areas of Downtown Los Angeles. My angelic team is very proud of me.

Freya reactivates the positive Egyptian royalty aspects of another timeline; the gifts, the knowing, the wisdom (Radhaa hears "Wisdom keeper"). I share with Radhaa that Gene Keys 48: Wisdom is my Pearl sphere, the center sphere in my prosperity sequence, which moves from the shadow of inadequacy to the highest essence of wisdom; and, it is through the path of resourcefulness. And I acknowledge Gene Keys 11: Light is my Vocation & Core sphere transforming all my suffering from the shadow of obscurity to the most profound potential of light, and to motivate me to excel in life by way of idealism. Everything is lining up. In this timeline, my gifts, wisdom, and what I am here to help others remember or reactivate are coming online, helping them remember themselves through the Gene Keys. This work is significant, bringing this foundation back online. Bringing these codes back online. Radhaa is a divine witness.

This part of my Egyptian royal lineage within me has now been reactivated, downloading it back into my consciousness. "Packets are going to start to activate." Radhaa sees an Egyptian man who is royal. "He might be in your life right now, helping him reactivate his royalness, helping them remember, and for those, I am here to serve. We're here to be embodied to bring heaven on Earth; in our embodiment, we are holders of these codes." She sees Goddess Isis of Divine Rebirth and now sees more Goddesses coming forward in my activation, Goddess Hathor of Divine Motherhood, Goddess Bastet of Divine Protection, Goddess Ma'at of Divine Truth, Justice & Cosmic Order. All were letting me know they stood alongside me in support. I could feel their presence coming forward, receiving chills from head to toes. I could feel my soul fragments coming online is the term used for integrating into me. It felt like I was receiving an icy cold intravenous fluid in the center top of my crown chakra.

Now that I have taken the time to meditate, I imagine myself as a pillar of light wherever I roam, connecting the light of the heavens above with Earth. Bringing in the warm golden light through the crown down into my solar plexus, then sending the rainbow light around me in all directions, in the form of a glowing, cosmic star. I can feel a warm love and light sensations arising in my heart, cells, and then in each of my chakras, activating the codes of remembering and the rainbow bridge that many ancient sacred texts speak of. From my heart center to Earth's crystalline core, activating our rainbow-like Merkabahs, I am raising my vibration and the planet's vibration.

"I am one with the Earth. The Earth and myself are one mind."
– Dr. José Argüelles, PhD

Pillar of Fire

The sun has now set on the Pacific Coast, and I am facing the East to perform an ancient purifying Vedic yajña (fire ritual or ceremony). Precisely at sunset, I recite a mantra to preserve the sun overnight. Next, I place two offerings into the fire that burn specific organic elements within the vessel. The sound vibrations of my voice infuse in the upside-down copper pyramid and ash that thrust up into the atmosphere. Finally, I stay calm and sit quietly with the dancing fire in meditation with a pure heart full of love and gratitude until the fire extinguishes itself.

This fire ceremony is called Agnihotra; Agni means fire, and hotra means healing. The agency of fire tunes to the specific circadian biorhythm of sunrise and sunset. It is not religious, and it is a peaceful practice I share with my son and an energy ritual that provides actual healing results. When performed, Agnihotra can reduce stress, bring greater clarity of thought, give one increased energy level and improve overall health. It purifies water resources, nourishes plant life, and neutralizes harmful radiation and pathogenic bacterias (Koch, 2004).

The pyramid symbolism, the Greek word "pyr" means fire, and "mid" means middle, so we have "Fire In The Middle." The pyramid acts as a receiver and transmitter of subtle energies radiating into the atmosphere. Creating a channel, or "pillar of energy from the fire" as I like to call it, reaching up about 7 miles north like a pillar into the biosphere, where the layer of particles with nutrients and pranic energy or vital life force is drawn down through this channel towards the pyramid.

As I purify the atmosphere, I absorb the healing energies around the pyramid. It purifies and cleans the space element from negative vibrations, replacing them with positive ones. Negative vibrations can be from the subtle pollutants arising from bad thoughts, bad words, bad deeds, and negative emotions from other people, which may cause harm. Any thought, comment, or feelings entertained by a person becomes a vibration and settle in the space. One of the main reasons I spend my nights and grand risings in the AM (no longer in "mourning") is healing the atmosphere as the healed atmosphere heals me.

I am honored and grateful to be a holder of the Pillar of Light with the Goddess Activations™ and share such a powerful practice with my family. To heal our environment and support everyone who lives within a mile radius of the center resonance point. This point includes healing the Downtown Los Angeles Financial District.

Freya is with me every step of the way as we link to higher realms of the galactic cosmos, spiritual guides, archangels, ancestors, and our planets' ancient wisdom keepers and beings. They sing and dance together through me, reminding me to have fun. Reassuring that without me, they would not have a voice or have a way of communicating, thus creation could not be expressed. I have the Divine knowledge to help others through my spiritual guidance and process. Knowing that I hold all of the wisdom of the entire Universe in the center portal of my heart. Love is all there is. I am on track.

Radhaa has now activated my Pillar of Light, expanding my vibration. I now commit to stepping into Freya's energy and operating only at that higher energetic level, looking forward to my power and strength. It was clear that I was heaven and Earth in pure expression, and I am and will continue to be a conduit for the light of the heavens to the Earth. I am a seeress. I am a rainbow bridge.

"I am a pillar of light."

With Love & Gratitude, Y'Shell

Saying:

"In today's world, both men and women need motherhood, the nurturing motherly feeling, the feminine energy. By receiving this energy, it will make them independent and free."

~ Mata Amritanandamayi

Y'SHELL ESTA

~ CONTRIBUTING WRITER ~

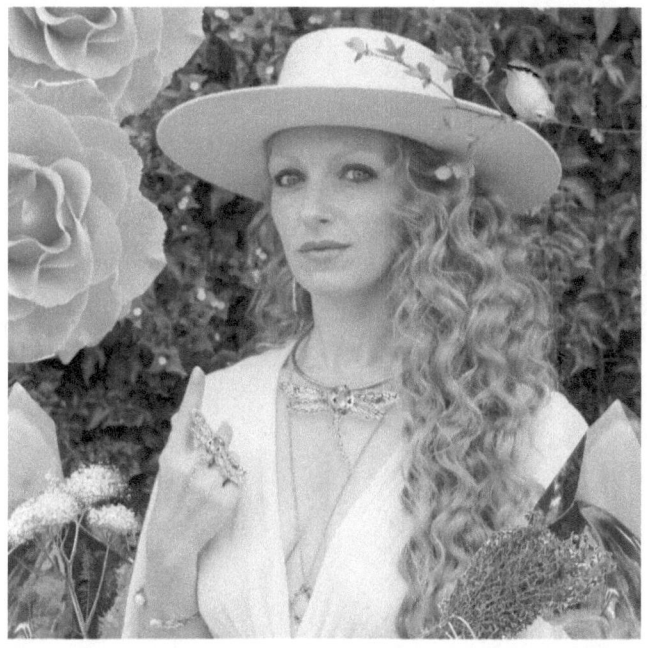

Activating Awareness through Love, Gratitude & Consciousness

Y'Shell Esta is a Gene Keys Guide, Pathfinder, Wisdom Keeper, Cosmic Warrior, and a Creative Collaborative Artist, Writer, and Producer. As a collaborative writer for the transformational book "Pillars of Light: Stories of Goddess Activations™" Y'Shell shares her experience through her Goddess Activation™ for the goddess archetype of Freya and an end to feminine pain of old paradigms, transforming her journey into a triumphant holder as a Pillar of Light located in sunny southern California.

As a Gene Keys Guide, she helps others find the information they are looking for through embracing real-life challenges and breakthroughs while guiding them towards their higher purpose. She also offers her own unique Gene Keys Relationship Equivalent readings and Individual Equivalent readings based on your personalized Hologenetic Profiles. Y'Shell has recently launched "Activation Aloud: #EvolveTheSpecies" an apparel line which are designs inspired by the Gene Keys.

Additional work has been as a video co-producer for the music video "I/O" by Mikuak Rai, both the "ALIGN with EARTH" mini-series leading to "ALIGN with EARTH, A Celebration of Regenerative Arts & Culture" live broadcast event on Earth Day 2021, presented in partnership with EarthDay.org and UNIFY. She is an additional vox on the hi-resonance track "Galactivation" from the album SIRIUS CODES: The Great Conjunction, written, produced, and performed by Mystic Column (MC2).

You can visit her online at https://shellyesta.com.

CHAPTER 14

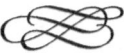

GREEN TARA GODDESS ACTIVATIONS™

Michelle Lopez

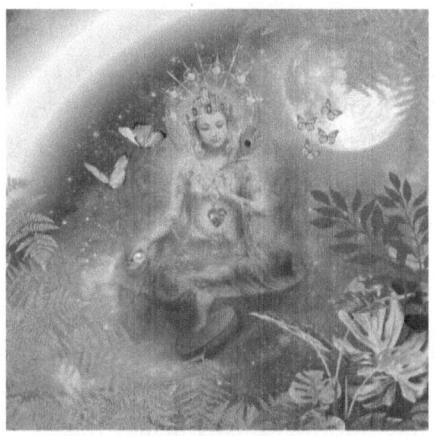

My Power is in my Innocence

Goddess Activations™ - At first glance, one may question the nature of this work. What is all the fuss about? Why do spiritual communities put so much emphasis on "The Goddess?" Is this worship? Is this feminism? One might think of this departure from mainstream thought of God as a male anthropomorphic being as blasphemous and heretical. However, truth is stranger than fiction. I know this supposed blasphemy to be one of the most honored and treasured secrets of the Earth's mystery teachings. As we enter the age of grace and a return to innocence, it is time to re-embrace this sacred mystery.

The truth is we are all birthed from a feminine womb. The universe herself is always birthing new worlds, and ours is no different,"As above, so below, as within so without." The ancient hermetic wisdom states. We are a microcosm of divinity, a fractalization of the source. Each Goddess teaching reaches into a lost and hidden part of ourselves, waiting to be discovered. We all carry the Goddess Codes™. They just have to be activated. These codes are part of our sacred heart, the carrier of feminine wisdom. A wisdom that has been suppressed for much of linear time on this Earth. The divine feminine is flooding the planet with light to heal and restore a broken and imbalanced world.

One of the earliest civilizations before recorded ancient civilizations was Lemuria. It is my understanding that Lemuria was energetically feminine. Their time and expression were much more crystalline and watery. They spent their days dancing, celebrating, and honoring all creation. Life was simple, innocent, and they were full of light. This civilization was the mother of all creation. Before we fell in our expression and fell out of balance with the masculine that was later to come.

So when the opportunity arose to be a part of the Goddess Activations™, I considered the power of all of these Goddesses coming together as a collective to share this heart wisdom. I felt it as immediate heart energy and the potential for portal creation to aid in the ushering of this feminine wisdom. It's a great honor to be a part of that. Each Goddess here in this book is a living crystal carrying ancient codes activated during this transition and change on Earth. Collectively, we are ushering humanity through yet another Stargate.

I met Radhaa quite organically several years ago when I was in the first Awakening Starseeds Book. One thing that drew me to work with Radhaa and Radhaa Publishing was Radhaa's connection to Quan Yin. I felt our work together was guided by this Goddess, and it was no accident that we would meet up at some point. I, too, had felt Quan Yin's guiding hand in my life. I felt an immediate understanding and connection with Radhaa on a soul level. It's like, "Oh, I see you, and I get you!" Her laugh, smile, and appreciation for beauty resonated with my own. I see Radhaa as a transmuter of energies.

The Goddess has reached into me in many ways since my awakenings.

Many months before, after moving into a new apartment positioned over a beautiful green park filled with trees, I received a synchronistic sign from Green Tara! Upon moving into this new place, I decided the large window in my bedroom overlooking this park needed some extra sparkle, so I hung some beveled crystals I owned in the window. I owned these old pieces of glass for many years and never realized the beautiful rainbows they created until then. Each afternoon when the sun would shine through the window, there would be beautiful rainbows dancing all over my room! So I decided to add to the effect, and I purchased a beautiful crystal beveled paperweight to add to my prayer altar. I set it right next to a statue of Green Tara, Goddess Lakshmi, Buddha, candles, and dried roses on my altar. I placed a dried rose on Green Tara. Those energies blend so well together, I thought!

With this particular crystal, the sun would shine through at just the right angle, and there would be little miniature rainbows everywhere! One afternoon, I came out of the bathroom to see Green Tara and a vibrant green fractal of light dazzling and shining so brightly! It's as if she was winking at me and trying to get my attention. So beautiful and radiant, I thought! I sat and pondered at this vibrant, pure, and radiant green light frequency emanating. I took note of it and a photo and forgot about it.

It all made sense when it came time for my activation. Green Tara is akin to the female buddha, and some see Quan Yin and Tara as the same energy. Quan Yin can come through as Tara. I believe they are sisters! Green Tara already let me know she wanted to work with me months before my activation with Radhaa.

In Sanskrit, Tara is the radiant one, the shining star. In the Gaelic tradition, it means "hill," which is associated with an elevated place, a place reserved for royalty. In yet other traditions, it means "star" but is associated with the ocean as in Stella Maris or "Star of the Sea" connecting to Venus/Aphrodite and Mother Mary to this energy.

Green Tara is also loosely associated with Terra, which means Earth, hence another association with Gaia Sophia, a lush, living, breathing planet composed mostly of water and becoming a shining and radiant star within the Cosmos as she ascends. Sophia represents the organic within us all and our innocence. In the Hindu tradition, she is Tara Devi, associated with the fierceness of Kali and Durga. Tara is a blending of all of the energies I had considered for this activation. She would be the perfect Goddess to work with.

Water is the bridge between worlds, and I am a soul in between worlds. It is a return to my innocence, much like the time when we were part of Lemuria. We were organic beings, relishing and reveling in our purity, sensuality, and innocence. We were like jellyfish in an ocean free of gravity and time. There was no need for anything other than our own beingness and joy. We are all to embark on this journey home, but not all will at this time of ascension. So here I am, taking the first step out of my comfort zone on this journey home. It is my soul reclaiming her Sovereignty. No more reincarnation, I am an incarnating being, and I honor my own free will and claim what my birthright is! My soul recognizes itself now.

Goddess Activations™ with Radhaa

Radhaa created a very beautiful and sacred space for my activation. She used her inner vision to call in my team. It was the enchanted realm and the elementals that came through. She picked up on benevolent green dragon energy as well. They were all holding space for me. Quan-yin came through as well, as she has been working with my higher self for a while. The energy of this space was very safe and calm. I felt a tremendous amount of energy in all my upper chakras, particularly around my crown and third eye. Radhaa ascertained that I had built a wall around my heart chakra. She called in the Goddess Green Tara to pour energy into me and fill my heart with this energy. Radhaa felt that my heart walls formed due to the grief and pain I experienced from the past. Some of it was old pain, some of it not so old. So we worked on that energy. She filled me up with liquid green light.

Green Tara collapsed all the old timelines. These timelines consisted of persecution and betrayal energy when I was not accepted as an herbal healer. I was a very bright light and good at my craft in that life. However, it was not safe for me. I was removed from that game.

We discussed the ancestral energies present. Much of my experience in this lifetime had much to do with these ancestral energies. These controllers made themselves known to me this past many years and to Radhaa during our session. Under normal circumstances, I feel these controllers who manipulate our reality in the form of ancestral karma largely go unnoticed by the collective. They are internal energies based on the DNA lineages we inherit. However, because I have done so much work to claim my Sovereignty, they are no longer unnoticed, nor are they quiet.

She saw this timeline ending in flames. She determined this was remnants of an old timeline, and these dark wizards are trying to hook into my pain body and continue to create harm as they did in the past. We cleared the timelines.

These ancestral energies came to me as karmic debt that I did not create. Through soul contract revocations I have been practicing, it is the end of the road for them. They will not be coming with me when I make my full transition. It is the birthing of a new timeline free from interference. Radhaa said that the Goddess was crowning me in this activation and put a pearl in my 3rd eye. This pearl formed through many lifetimes of experiences that took me further away from my original innocence. The pearl is a reminder of the beautiful masterpiece being created. These experiences are no longer necessary to move forward on the journey.

A few days had passed after the activation when the layers of this onion began to unravel. Seemingly out of the blue, I felt triggered by life circumstances that showed up, and I felt the emotions come up somewhat uncontrollably. I began to shed many tears, and once the floodgates opened, they did not stop for the remainder of the day. When the first layer of this onion came off, it was very painful. So much of the pain I had been holding was being released. I had a good friend keep me company during this process, and we talked most of the afternoon. I realized that Green Tara was activating me for an even deeper love and compassion for myself. It almost came with a bit of fierceness. She helped me understand that it was okay to feel this fierce love for myself as my soul had endured much.

I felt pretty tender after the first layer. Ouch! That layer was painful, and it was much like having a bandaid ripped off! I followed up my activation with Radhaa with a full moon parasite cleanse, releasing more of the onion-like layers. The synchronicity seemed fitting. During this time, the thing that hit home with me was that everything I have had to endure in my life experience was beautifying and polishing me into that beautiful pearl.

It is a return to innocence. By innocence, I mean the original state of the soul as it existed before the density and karma got a hold of it. We are all born innocent and hold a divine spark within that is pure and untouched. Green Tara helped me see that this is the first step in the transition back home, and the pearl represents that.

As a soul, I understand that I likely have played every role there is to play on this planet. It no longer makes any difference who I was. It is who I am today that counts. There is no hierarchical order in this game of Earth life and no winners and losers. There is only a return to our original innocence. The gift of Green Tara has come through since my session with Radhaa, and she is paving the way for my journey home.

There have been times in my life, especially after my awakening, where I realized how naive I may have been in my life, how trusting I was of others, and how so often I only saw people in their goodness. When I did see their shortcomings, I tended to overlook them, considering them less important than the potential I saw. "Don't fall in love with potential!" The saying goes! What was happening here is I was projecting my desirable traits onto others and not using my discernment to see what was not meant for me. It's a part of myself that I hid or disowned.

"Why am I so trusting and naive?" Green Tara helped me to see that this is not a negative trait. It is a gift. However, this gift must also be coupled with discernment! I also became aware that I had also developed a distrust of others in my effort to be discerning. The gift is understanding that I embody that innocence myself. It is the recognition of the true soul essence. Many of us tend to project our good qualities onto others instead of recognizing them in ourselves. Of course, I have an ego, a persona, and limitations of earthly existence. Still, as I move forward, I can continue to progress in my embodiment of the soul and authentic expression.

I compare this 'original innocence' to my work with children and as a voice for the animals. Children are naturally authentic, and so is the animal kingdom. The animals teach us how to act naturally and work cooperatively in groups. The animal kingdom maintains diversity while maintaining a delicate balance present in nature. They are the ultimate teachers for how we can live authentically as humans. Children learn by playing. They have a natural propensity for joy. They often lose this as they grow into adulthood because it is "schooled" out of them. It is the beginning of the loss of innocence. The amnesia within the culture takes over, and the innocence of the soul is eclipsed.

I have just mentioned working with children in the schools and being a voice for the animals. The wisdom they bring is the bridgework Tara is helping me with. Tara is often seen with a rainbow around her. She can connect with every ray of colored expression on this Earth. It is the 8th ray. I see this 8th ray as the bridging of spirit and matter. Green Tara is activating me to continue to be a guide and teacher to others by merging higher concepts into the here and now on this Earth. She is activating me as a translator for the concepts that those humans awakening and those not yet awakened to comprehend. She activates me, and I activate others to see their full human potential. That is the domino effect this work has on humanity. I am helping them to individuate and maintain their divine innocence. The children of this New Earth will need leaders to help them maintain their purity of spirit.

Our innocence is our connection to Earth, to our source. This connection is one of the most powerful tools available to us. I am personally claiming this connection with the help of Green Tara and many other of my higher self celestial guides. This connection to the source is helping me to birth a new timeline of my creation and is untouched by any outside interference. It is the path of Dharma where I become an emanation of source as a conduit rather than a recipient of karma. I am in the process of creation and alchemy. Could you not ask me to explain the magic? To do that is to ask me to engage the logical, linear mind. There is no logic in this expression. That is why it is pure and untainted. I base this future timeline on my faith, trust, and knowing that a piece of me already exists there. It is something my soul planned long before I came to this Earth.

This divine innocence is present within me because of my connection to source-the divine mother and the divine father. We all have this divine blueprint within us that is there for reclaiming when our souls are ready for it. It gives birth to the Sophia Christ child within. As I reclaim my divinity, I reclaim my power. "There is Power in my Innocence." When the mythological Eve entered the Garden of Eden, she didn't know she was naked or that any aspect of life could not be experienced or tasted. It wasn't until the world told her she was naked and forbidden to taste the tree of knowledge that things got complicated. That is the journey of karma we have been on ever since.

As I sit here and write this, I ask myself, why is this even possible? The ability to heal, reclaim our birthright, shift timelines, and return to innocence is not something spiritual traditions even speak of? In the past, you would have to meditate in a cave for a lifetime to balance karmas and spend lifetimes trying to understand life's mysteries, and that is if you were on a spiritual path. It is all possible because we live in a time of grace and ascension. The Goddesses are here to restore balance to this broken world. We are ascending to a world of peace and wholeness. We need to do our part, be of service, and love others as they are.

I am grateful to have had the session with Radhaa and honored to be activated in the Green Tara energy. As I step forward on this ascension journey, I am now empowered with the power of my innocence. Green Tara is aiding me in the embodiment of my soul essence. I have a ways to go, but I am on my way. Stepping into the unknown, untethered.

> My heart surrenders
> An empty vessel
> Her nectar fills me
> The walls
> They were erected long ago
> She reminds me they are no
> Longer necessary to guard this
> Precious heart
> The medicine witch, the amazon,
> The refugee
> They don't matter
> What matters is who she is now
> Swept away on a sea of ecstasy
> She returns with her elixir
> They are the stirrings of a Goddess lying dormant
> Like a volcano, she rises
> Ashes and fire would seem to destroy everything in its wake
> It does not! Instead, the ash
> Creates a rich soil for seeds to grow
> The Goddess reigns once again
> Life grows where there once was none.
> Only she can stir the hearts of men
> Who have only known war

Only she can breathe life into women.
Who has been slaves to a race of people with amnesia?
Only she can nurture the children of
Tomorrow, the future belongs to them
Children with free will
She takes her place alongside her King
God and Goddess, the bridal chamber is ready
Enter the Great Mystery.

MICHELLE LOPEZ

~ CONTRIBUTING WRITER ~

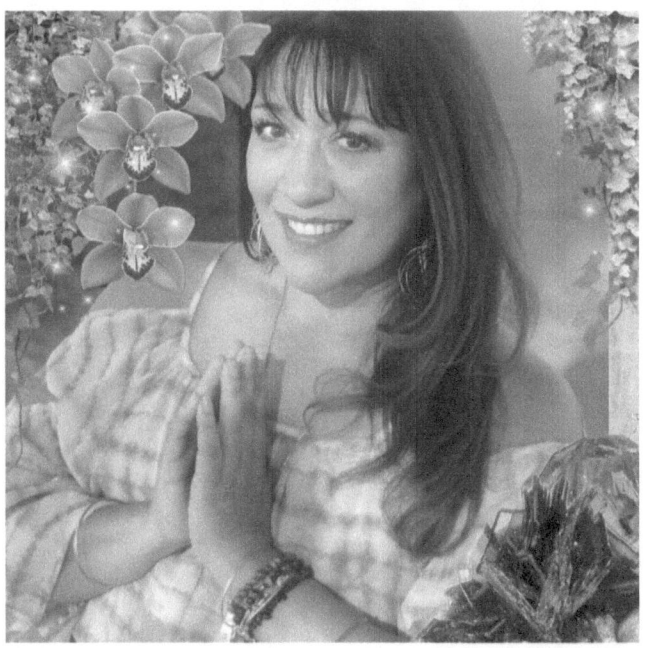

Michelle Kearney Lopez is a holistic healer specializing in divination and reiki energy healing. She utilizes astrology, oracle and tarot cards, crystals, and sound tools to bring awareness to areas of the psyche that need healing. She is also an elementary school teacher, children's book author, and children's yoga and mindfulness instructor. Her lightworker mission is to bridge, work with the human heart template, and activate others into their transformation and healing and, ultimately, their ascension. Michellekearneylopez.com

Saying:

"The Divine Feminine lives within you, within me, within us all. For the past few thousand years, she has been repressed, cast into the shadows, and left without a safe place to fully express herself and her gifts. But she is on the rise. She is slowly waking up and returning to us all. Women (and men) around the world are hearing her call."

~ Shani Jay

CHAPTER 15

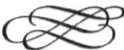

CASSANDRA GODDESS ACTIVATIONS™

Lori Santo

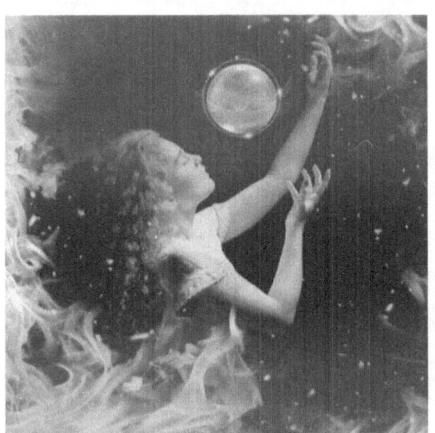

My Goddess Activations™ encounter with Radhaa was incredibly powerful, astute, and immediately seeded deeply within my body. I have worked with many archetypes over a couple of decades, yet few deeply call to me for fully embodied integration of how some of the darker, more misunderstood archetypes do; Cassandra, Kali, Sekhmet, and Lillith, name a few.

I am from a historical lineage of deep and severe generational trauma and abuse: emotional, mental, physical, sexual (including rape), and spiritual, and it is saturated with curses, predators, and distortions of all types. From my early childhood, I knew that I came to change the course of history in my ancestry and my bloodline past, present, and future, along with the insanity inherent within it. I came into the world equipped with a profound, holy responsibility to stop the severe abuses in their tracks. I was an awkward child, shy and deeply sensitive, withdrawn, terrified of the predators that surrounded me, and afraid of my power from the start. I was very tender about protecting my ferocity in the face of so much surrounding familial trauma, and I was aware just how hungry they all were for my power. I was the third of six children, the first girl, and before I was old enough to understand what was happening (age 3) consciously, my siblings were being hit, kicked, slapped, screamed at, and I was being molested. Regularly. My molester didn't stop until I was 15.

Enter the Dragons. My highly creative, keenly imaginative artist self was my constant companion; she was a wizard of high intelligence, an ancient, sovereign creatrix, and a magician of epic prowess in her own right. Before the age of five, I remember calling upon wizards, trolls, fairies, witches, elves, dragons, and miracles to help me in my enchanted wonderment to become a force that was larger than life. My feminine Merlin, to ward off all the evil, dark forces within my fortress. Little did I know then how my brilliant imagination was seeding my very becoming. I spent all of my childhood, into my adolescence, in a well-developed, self-created world of angels, guardians, magic, and miracles, and was praying to my Creator from the time I could speak. I was slaying dragons and curses, I was well armored against the onslaught of predators and distorted perversions of all types in all dimensions, seen and unseen, and it was unrelenting work to be the warrior and protector of so many younger siblings and cousins. I lived for their safety and believed it was possibly the sole reason for my existence. By the time I turned 16, I had fallen in love with becoming a young maiden. A sexy, hot, sensual young woman on fire, my mother finally left my egregiously dangerous father and turned our lives in a mind-boggling spin in a new direction, and, well, every single thing changed. While I began to experience my newfound freedom as a teenager, now liberated from the abusive control of my raging father, I was simultaneously becoming intimately acquainted with the dark undercurrent pulling me deep down into the abyss of terror with all of the unspoken abuses and prolific violations, never spoken.

Enter my beginning path in therapy, which I engaged in from that ripe age of 16 and continued for many decades to follow. My childhood had been consumed by the dangerously abusive, neglectful, mentally imbalanced adults surrounding my life en masse, and I had never uttered a word to a single soul about any of it until then. I had so many years of my flooded nervous system in overload and belief systems that were utterly insane, and shame was my strongest ally. My life had never been my own, and I was deeply afraid of myself and all of my hidden secrets. I had become agoraphobic, and I could not speak. That lasted for well over a year. I soon became a falling-down drunk and consumed any drugs and dealers I could get my hands on for years. I was the consummate addict. I spent two significant stays in mental institutions for nervous breakdowns in my late twenties and thirties, when the onslaught of all of my fragmented, sharded-off traumas (and sub-personalities) came to greet me as I deepened my commitments in sobriety, therapy, and spiritually oriented healing modalities. It took years of doing the very deep immersions with spiritual and physical healers, ministers, psychotherapists, priests performing exorcisms, gurus, medications, rehabs, twelve-step programs, hospital stays, all of it before I began to recognize the absolute profundity of how much power had been siphoned from me and took me out of myself altogether. It took decades for me to begin coming home to myself, healing so much trauma, rage, and madness, integrating back into my body. There were many years of writing, journaling, healing, exercising (including becoming a marathon runner), really great and appropriate types of trauma therapy, releasing layer by layer, the seemingly insurmountable wounds to my Soul splitting completely away from me, as my trembling body feared Her coming back into Being. There are many reasons for a powerful warrior on a deeply Sacred spiritual journey. For me, most of my seasons were spent in battle, defending everyone around me. I had no idea how to do it until it was a new season when they all moved on and no one left to defend me. Let alone how to even be with me. As a highly sensitive, empathic, astutely emotional woman, my experience is that there is a predominant culture in the coaching and self-help industries that are saturated in "love and light," "raising your vibration." platitudes that have done tremendous and significant damage to sensitive beings like me who have been through life-altering trauma. Hell, personality-altering levels of trauma. As a life coach and an artist, I am fiercely devoted to changing these highly toxic, surface delusional teachings. Love and Light cannot exist without the depth and dimensions of darkness.

In 2016, I took the highly courageous step of coming out of the proverbial shadows. I took the stage and performed a version of my story to the world. As an introvert who carried enough shame for all of us, this was an epic and heroic move, and it took every ounce of my bravery. It changed me in ways unimagined, and I have never experienced anything quite so powerful in my life. Another step in my evolution into my true, raw power.

Enter Radhaa!

Radhaa and I met in 2016, working together in taking the stage, and from the moment we met, I knew I had to know her more intimately. I resonated so powerfully with her; she felt like a lightning rod and a tuning fork, and I was fascinated to discover what I was tuning into about her. As our friendship blossomed over time and I experienced her Goddess Activation work, everything became clear.

Radhaa is a gifted Seer with laser powers of mastery in her perceptions of the deep darkness. More importantly, her skill at slaying within it is compelling, and it is felt in the body as she moves with precision, downloading her insights of the content of your Higher Truth.

Enter Cassandra

As Radhaa weaved Cassandra's guidance throughout my activation, the distinctions of Cassandra's influence were clear and direct. Cassandra was a highly misunderstood prophet, and no one believed her insights (all of which came to be). Her brilliance was not recognized until after her death. She was a mystic, a seer, and she carried powerful profound psychic powers. I feel unusually resonant to Cassandra ~ it was natural for me to embody her; she is a kindred spirit, very much a part of myself I didn't realize was missing. She is larger than life force, and her messages landed in me in the deepest crevices. I now understand both the ferocity and the fire that escorted me into the world with me as my true allies.

Cassandra came to support and guide me in shifting my consciousness as the layers of demonic curses were peeled from me and my lineage. At the same time, Radhaa did her skillful, technically astute reading of my inner landscapes.

Cassandra and Radhaa together is a once-in-a-lifetime experience, and it didn't take long before the two organically became the same. Radhaa had full command, and the presence of Cassandra's power was felt in Radhaa's voice. I sensed the gentle release of generations of dark entities, curses, karmic imprints, distortions, and unnatural implants that I have battled with for decades. Together, they carried epic prowess, and the experience was stunning to my spirit. She also reminded me of my arsenal of superpowers that have laid dormant, awaiting my full presence and arrival.

Together, they took me on an epic remembrance of my wholeness, as I was reacquainted and integrated with my mega guardians and archetypes, namely Quan Yin, Archangel Michael, and my Enchanted Self (my Feminine Merlin).

Next, Radhaa masterfully weaved in all of my early life companions – and magical memories of my devoted, strong dragons, wizards, fairies, trolls, witches, elves, and miraculous guides at my sides, while I quietly celebrated it all feeling like Home as she continued to work. She reactivated my Ancient, Enchanted Self back into a larger-than-life force. I made a quantum leap in time, and I was aware of my High Caliber Divine Creatrix, the Eternal Self, as she continued to cast her spells of Truth.

Radhaa's accuracy is stunning. My unshakeable inner knowing has been seeded once again. That there is no doubt. My power is back, and it's really big, as it contains so much of the warrior aspects needed now to resurrect. Conscious shifts are necessary for our ongoing evolution collectively. I am divinely protected, guided, directed, and informed. Radhaa and Cassandra removed and cleared all of my inner debris and density and simultaneously reactivated and realigned my mystical, prophetic aspects.

I am taking the liberty of sharing a poem activated after my time with Radhaa and Cassandra. In honor of all who are battling big things deeply alone, many of whom don't get the privilege of Conquering them.

This poem is created for the brave, courageous warrior women I know, doing the hard work on behalf of all of us, especially those who rage and burn in silence and the predators who tried to destroy us. I want to talk about archetypes and warriors.

It is to Radhaa and Cassandra, and I offer my greatest gratitude for the Role in my Resurrection.

LORI SANTO
~ CONTRIBUTING WRITER ~

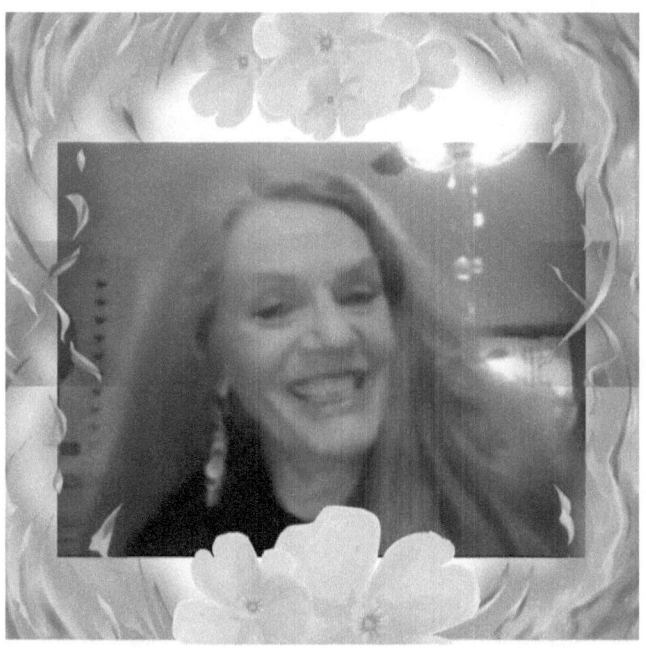

Lori is a mother to a teenage son, a visionary artist, poetic storyteller, certified life coach, and a passionate writer. The latter's work is devoted to the Sacred, Wild Feminine and healing of trauma and sexual abuse. Lori brings her poetry and storytelling to public stages. She has been featured in three best-selling books. Her research and study over decades include Ancient Wisdom, Mysticism, Metaphysics, and Buddhism. In 2001, she took refuge in the Hanmi Lineage under Living Buddha Dechan Jueren (Chinese esoteric Buddhist Master Yu).

She worked directly with Master Yu as his disciple for 1-1/2 years before returning to Beijing. Visit: www.lorisanto.com

CHAPTER 16

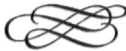

MOTHER MARY GODDESS ACTIVATIONS™

Kory Muniz

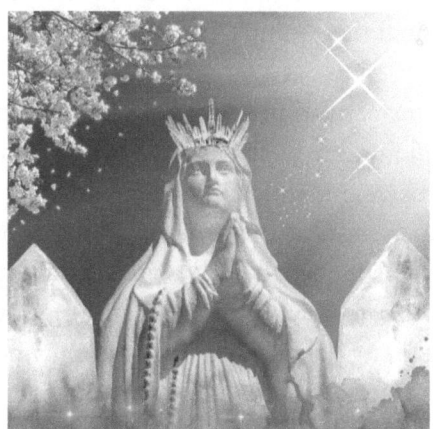

Being a Reiki Master/Teacher, I meditate and have utilized several modalities of emotional healing throughout the years and have received much healing; however, nothing has affected me in such a mind-blowing way as my Goddess Activations™ with Radhaa.

"And in my hour of darkness, she is standing right in front of me, Speaking words of wisdom, Let it be." - *Paul McCartney*

Goddess Activations™ with Radhaa

Sometimes you meet someone, and your soul recognizes them. It was how I felt the first time I met Radhaa in the early 2000s. I was immediately drawn to her magnetic smile and warm aura. Beauty was in every corner of her lovely home, and the glowing energy I felt I knew was there from her being. I knew that our connection was divinely led, and we would be friends and somehow work on a project together.

Her insightfulness and loving spirit permeate all that surrounds her.

Knowing Radhaa through the years and watching her unfold into the beautiful butterfly and Goddess she is today has been truly a blessing. I am so happy to see the world embrace her as she continues to inspire others to open their minds, hearts, and wings so that they, too, can soar.

At the time of my activation session, I was a hot mess, as they say. Dealing with rebuilding my business after over a year of lockdowns in California, I have been empathic all my life and always had a knowing beyond my life experiences at the time. I had many premonitions, and I would tell others about what I saw, but I would get in trouble for doing so. I retreated into a spiritual closet until I gave birth to my son at thirty-five. Something just burst open within my heart, and I knew I had to get back on track. The search for answers continued. Still, I had many questions and few answers. My Goddess Activation™ with Radhaa has answered my deepest quest.

Before our session, Radhaa asked me if I would like to work with a specific Goddess, and I told her that I work with the Eastern Goddess of Compassion Quan Yin. As we settled into our time together, her warm, loving voice and energy lulled me into complete comfort and safety. Feelings I haven't felt in a while. I have been attempting to process big energetic changes happening but not exactly understanding my part in all of it.

I felt like all things good were just within my reach, but some blockages around me were stopping me from experiencing it. I could feel it, and it was palpable. But I was STUCK.

Deep feelings of sadness, anger, frustration, rage, grief, inconsolable torment, betrayal and impending doom rose within my spirit.

After being invited to step into a sacred space, Radhaa asked me to share my intentions. Then she asked me why I was drawn to Quan Yin. As I was answering her, I could feel the energies surrounding me becoming lighter. I felt the need to be open to any other Goddesses who wished to step in during this activation.

With three cleansing breaths together, we were on our journey. As I breathed down into my womb and exhaled any stagnant energy as Radhaa had instructed, she invited me to join her in being in the heart of the creator of all that is. She called upon all of my ascendant Angels, masters and guides, ancestors that assisted me on my journey.

The very same I call in when doing a Reiki session.

We touched bases on how I was feeling. I felt as if I was being embraced in a very motherly way. Without the fear of being judged. An experience I hadn't felt since I was sixteen and lost my mother to Breast Cancer.

I felt free from the 3D stuff as Radhaa put it as she giggled with me. Her lightheartedness and genuine caring for me were obvious in her giggle. I could fully breathe.

As Radhaa brought Quan Yin into our space, I welcomed her, feeling her energy. Radhaa was telling me that she was seeing Mother Mary as well. She stood in front of me while Quan Yin supported my back.

It was shocking and brought back a couple of memories when I sought spiritual healing with bodywork practitioners who told me that Jesus was standing at my crown chakra. At the time, it just passed through my consciousness, not really thinking about it much and differently not exploring why. And now Mother Mary was asking permission through Radhaa to work with me. As I tried to figure out my connection with Mother Mary, I was surprised that she would step forward to assist me, not being raised in a Christian household. Finally, Radhaa explained that Quan Yin is the Eastern version of Mother Mary.

Then I realized that one of my favorite places near me is Lake Shrine, a part of the ashram founded by Paramahansa Yogananda in 1950. It is a beautiful place to meditate and connect with the Divine. It is non-denominational, and the place I have always been most drawn to is an alcove with a bust of Mother Mary. So naturally, I will stop by to say hi and tell her how beautiful she is. But, as it turns out, she told me she was here for me.

I thought to myself, well, that made sense then. But wait, there's more.

As we continued, Radhaa told me that Mother Mary wanted to be with me in a stronger way. She's saying that there are some lifetimes that we need to clear, and some of them were lifetimes connected with the period where she lived.

Radhaa reminded me that Quan Yin was still with me, supporting me through this clearing at my back. I felt a deep sense of unconditional love and compassion as Quan Yin helped me stay in the feeling of wonder and openness.

The Divine Mother wanted me to know that I needed to clear things from that timeline shared with Jesus. Mother Mary shared that I walked with Jesus and saw what was happening to him. I was carrying a lot of trauma from that time. I was a woman, a healer, and I felt like a failure. I was feeling useless. Like there was nothing I could do to stop what was playing out before my eyes.

I felt frustrated, and no one would listen to me. And that was the timeline that most affected me in the here and now.

Say what?!

It hit me like a lightning bolt. Again, I was with my wellness business, trying to educate people on getting and staying healthy. Teaching how to use their thoughts to create their reality and use their discernment to see through the lies of the dark ones. And yet, so many have chosen to follow the darkness. Again!

I had been feeling the tug to give up, and it was mind-blowing that I heard Radhaa's voice those very words, "You felt like giving up!"

There was a war against the Divine as there is now. Where were the people who cared? Where were the people who wanted to stop it? Why is everyone just standing around and watching this happen? I felt defeated. We were bringing forth healing, empowering people. Why were we being sabotaged? I was and had been feeling inconsolable grief. And now, in 2021, why is it happening again?

The tears filled my eyes, and I had to take a moment to cry it out. These were my exact thoughts then and what I have been experiencing up until my Goddess Activations™.

As the timeline started to clear, I remembered when I managed a holistic massage clinic attached to The Touch Therapy Institute in Encino, California. I was making individual essential oils as Christmas gifts for my massage therapists, and one therapist was so happy with hers that she suggested that I make and sell them, and I told her that I would rather give them. She said she felt that idea came for me, not wanting to be followed as a seer. She asked if she could give me a reading as a sign of gratitude for the oil blend, and of course, I said, "yes, please."

I learned from this reading that I had been a spiritual leader in many lifetimes, and I had many followers, one particular incarnation. But, unfortunately, many were tortured and killed for following my teachings. The pain was too much to bear. Hearing this, I cried like never before. Deeper than when I lost my mother to cancer or my older sister's murder. It came from an unknown place, through my toes, and, like a volcano, gushed out my crown chakra. I knew what she was seeing was my truth.

YES, YES, YES!

During my activation, I remembered this once again, but this time I was armed to know that past experiences compounded my feelings of giving up and frustration. It was now easy to let go. The layers of the onion started to peel away.

When I was in my early twenties, I had an experience that I will never forget. While in West Hollywood, California, browsing through a metaphysical bookstore called the Bodhi Tree located on the well-known Melrose Avenue, a man who I did not know appeared next to me out of nowhere. He looked at me as if he knew me. All I could say was I didn't know him. He was standing extremely close to me, but I felt calm and safe in his presence for some reason. After gazing into my eyes, he said, "You don't know who you are, do you?" I didn't know what to say. So I said, "heck, I am here to learn how to figure that out!" Then he said, "You will." I looked down for a second being extremely shy and not knowing how to respond. When I looked up in his direction, he had vanished as quickly as he appeared. Did I experience an Angel or Divine messenger trying to help me remember this timeline?

What do you think?

I have always believed in Angels, but my baby boy brought that home. There are three experiences I will share with you. The first one was when I was nursing him. He nursed until two and a half years old and spoke full sentences by age two. Then, one day while nursing, he stopped. His whole face started to glow, and he was staring upward. I asked him what he was looking at, and his response made my hair stand on its end. His reply was, "GOD." He smiled, giggled then he went back to nursing. The second was just a few months later. We used to garden in our small backyard, and my son loved being out with the plants, butterflies, and bees. He ran into the house to get me because he saw Angels and wanted me to see them. The third was when he insisted on walking our very strong pitbull, Tiger. I explained that she was much stronger than him, and I didn't want him to get hurt. He was around four at this time. We negotiated, and he let us both hold her leash. Somehow the leash got tangled as we walked down the stairs that led to the alley, and he was knocked off his feet, but it looked as if someone was holding him by his back and pushing him forward, stopping him from hitting his head in the stairs.

You may ask what this has to do with the Goddess Activations™. Well, I will try to explain. I have had many experiences that brought doubt into my heart of the existence of the Divine and other beings like angels. I have been in and out, lacking true belief in my knowledge and without a foundation of self-awareness. That is until these experiences.

As I continued to see events play out through my third eye and heart chakras, Radhaa, with the guidance of Mother Mary, continued to be my tour guide through past lives, constantly checking in with me. Moving to a lifetime and trauma from Egypt. A place I have hoped to visit in this lifetime. The pyramids have been calling to me for as long as I can remember.

When a close friend, Simon, who I knew from first glance was part of my soul family, visited the great pyramids, all I wanted to do was hear how the frequencies affected him. He now has many Egyptian symbols and pyramids tattooed on his back. Since my Goddess Activation™, I realize we also have another connection.

In the next part of my session with Radhaa, I was off to Atlantis, where I was during its fall. It didn't surprise me at all. Though I fear being in the ocean and not seeing the shoreline, the ocean is my happy place. I have had visions of people falling into the ocean. People were running, screaming, crying, and drowning. Radhaa was there in that timeline as well. That's our heart connection? Were we a soul family? How many more coincidences could there be? How many connections? I could not go through any more past traumatic experiences.

MY GALACTIC FAMILY SHOWED UP when I thought I had seen and been told everything I needed to know. Radhaa felt they were Sirian and that I am a Sirian Starseed. Another truth bomb hit me like a ton of bricks.

I remember a visit to Disneyland when I was a teenager. They had a Star Wars ride. It was a visual and physical experience that took us through stars, planets, and galaxies. A sense of excitement filled my very being. It was almost orgasmic. I felt like I was going home. I endured the long line multiple times to experience it again and again. Another memory confirmed.

After unpacking this information, I searched online for Sirian Star Seeds, and what I read indicated my whole life, personality priorities, and life mission. So much more accurate than any astrology reading I have had.

What is a Sirian Starseed? From what I read, it is a rare type of star seed, reincarnated on Earth and encoded with Sirian DNA. Encrypted with codes ready to activate at a predetermined time. We are known as freedom and spiritual seekers. Deeply connected to Mother Earth, we are called Gaia's people. Anyone who knows me can contest those qualities embedded in who I am. Let's visit some other qualities, and I will explain how those pieces fit so well into my life. A vivid imagination-This one reminded me of most of my report cards saying, good student but often in her world. This was me, and it is also where Simon comes into play again.

As I stepped into the reality of what I was experiencing, I realized that I no longer am fearful. I have shown up time and time again. I have done enough. I have answered the call of the Divine, and it is time for me to find my bliss, reactivate the full healer within and release the feeling of impending doom.

I am now going to hold the line. My job is to raise my vibration and, in doing so, anchor it to the planet and all that live here. My chains are broken, vows of poverty severed, limitations ended, fears transmuted, mission understood and accepted.

"I now anchor this Pillar of Light. A grid is being created around the world. This grid activates the new earth templates and stabilizes it as the old Earth, and the old templates and the old programming are completely eroding. I understand my purpose and accept my mission in the here and now."

Listen to the little nudges you get. The more you listen, the more you will receive. We all become fearful at one time, but we don't have to stay in that vibration. It is never too late to find your divine center. We are not alone. "We are always supported, in always," as a dear friend and soul family member, Carolyn says.

I will never truly find the words of gratitude for this divine opportunity in my Goddess session by Radhaa so that I will end with a single word Radhaa repeated throughout my Goddess Activations™. "Simply Beautiful."

KORY MUNIZ
~ CONTRIBUTING WRITER ~

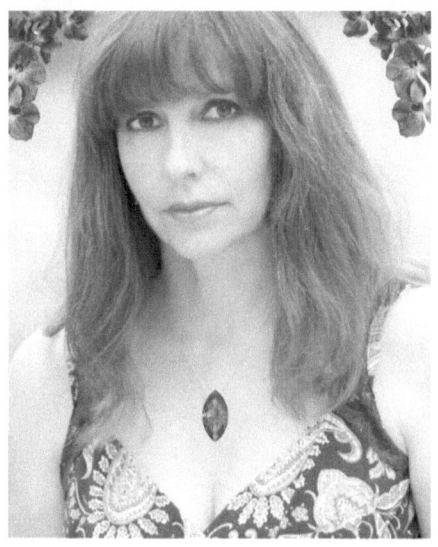

Intuitive since birth, Kory's healing journey with healing has been an ongoing process since childhood.

After the death of her beloved mother to breast cancer, she was determined to find ways to keep herself and loved ones healthy, knowing it is easier to maintain health than to take away dis-ease.

Although she has been doing energy work for over 30 years, her formal Reiki training started in 2002 under the guidance of a Reiki Master Teacher, Merel Sunde-Marschall. She continued her training with Merel until she reached the level of Reiki Master Teacher in the spring of 2004.

Kory also has The Touch Therapy Institute training in Crystal Healing, Color Therapy, and Clinical Aromatherapy. In addition to her healing practice, Kory is a gourmet raw food chef and educator.

Kory's mission is to connect the spirit of every being with the remembrance of unconditional love, healing, and self-empowerment.

Reach Kory at: VibrantHealthNaturally.com

CHAPTER 17

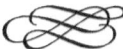

BRIGIT GODDESS ACTIVATIONS™

Michelle Casto

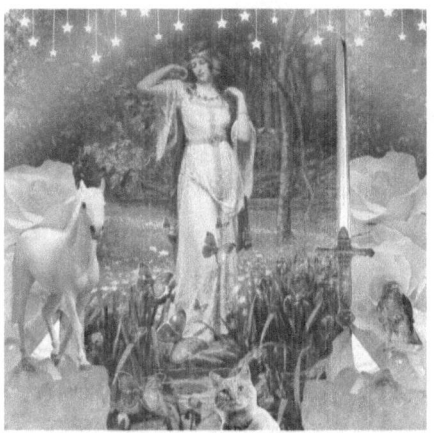

*H*ave you ever experienced the horrible feeling that you're trapped inside a bad dream? One where you are Aware enough to know that things are not as they should be, but try as you might, and you can't wake up out of it. It is a painful way to live, especially when you awaken and KNOW that you are a powerful creator and have divine power inside you.

It is my story, and I'd like to share how my Goddess Activations™ with Radhaa was a major turning point in my life.

Once upon a time, a sensitive, open-hearted little girl believed in magic, miracles, and that anything was possible.

She grew up in a family who didn't know how to love her unconditionally, were blind to her unique bright light, so she didn't receive the message that she was infinitely loved, gifted, talented, and worthy.

Her mother was especially cruel and seemed to take pleasure in siphoning her daughter's beautiful light and goodness. The little girl was an only child and felt like a prisoner with no chance for escape.

As she looked around this world, she couldn't understand why life felt so strange and how people could be mean and selfish. As an only child, she spent much of her young life connecting with nature, talking to animals, and reading books. She was exquisitely tuned into the MAGIC around her despite feeling sad, abused, and unloved an awful lot.

When she grew older, she lost some of her innocence and did what most people do, tried to find herself in achievements, goals, and romantic relationships. But when nothing would satisfy, she realized that something essential was amiss.

Even though she was aware, wise, and loving, she seemed stuck in a pattern of attracting one obstacle or disappointment after another. She saw other people letting bitterness overrun the sweetness of life, and she didn't want to follow them down that well-traveled road, and so she made a radical choice to heal her own heart.

Along the way, she discovered she was on a journey to discover her unique Destiny, and so she became a guide for other awakening earth angels.

Spell on Michelle

I was born empathic and tuned in to my surroundings, but instead of this sensitivity being understood and nurtured, it was neglected and even ridiculed. It was clear to me, even at a young age, that there was some invisible force that was out to take me down, especially if I started having "too much" pleasure, fun, success, and happiness.

There was a default program running on DON'T.

> Don't be too beautiful.
> Don't be too smart.
> Don't be too sexy.
> Don't speak your truth.
> And for God's sake, Don't be too much.

Gratefully, the Goddess wasn't going to let me settle for accepting outdated social mores regarding being a woman in the Great Awakening. After all, she had especially created me to do as I pleased and to enjoy the pleasures of life on Earth. I believe that Goddess Isis had placed a flame of remembrance in my SOUL that has compelled me forward to move beyond 'Don't' and all the other related dark mother and patriarchal dogma that was lodged in my psyche from the collective and ancestral consciousness.

As a teenager, I began fighting against my mother's control, criticism, and inability to honor my boundaries. In my early twenties, I consciously began working on myself with therapy and reading self-help books. As soon as I was able, I moved as far away as possible, thinking that would help. While the distance did allow me to live life more on my terms, *The Don't Be.... Happy, Successful, or Loved* program was surreptitiously installed and NOT to be easily over-written.

For most of my life (50 years), my heart felt so heavy and barren; the weariness felt like the weight of 1000's lives. I presume because this was the lifetime for me to Wake Up to honoring my divine feminine lineage.

Having a narcissistic and spiritually compromised mother and abandoning father made me feel like an orphan with no real family foundation to stand on. Not only did I long to find my true path in life, but I was quite desperate to get past the profound sense of despair that often was too much for one person to bear.

The Goddess kept nudging me forward. Even if her voice was faint as a whisper, I listened for guidance. Fortunately for me, I was a dedicated seeker who intuitively knew that I would eventually find and heal whatever was holding me back from following my bliss.

One of my first introductions with the Goddess Realm was a game called *Goddess Guide Me*. It was a multicolored box with beautiful, long-haired Goddesses on the cover. Inside, you could read corresponding cards that outlined individuals' wisdom as related to your inquiry. All I

had to roll the dice and pose a question. It was like a modern-day oracle, and I had high hopes that someone – hopefully a loving Goddess, was listening to my prayers.

In my 40's, I finally started to understand what it meant to be an empath and even wrote a book about it, *Heart Empowerment for Empaths*. The worst part about my upbringing was how much negativity and funkiness I had unconsciously absorbed from my mother.

Sadly, most, if not all, of my relationships suffered because I had unconsciously separated myself from love and success by buying into stories of shame and unworthiness.

Even though I knew I had been deeply wounded, no matter how much forgiveness or therapy work I did, I couldn't bring about my soul's liberation; until I experienced my Goddess Activations™.

The Goddess Activations™

The Goddess Activations™ work I did with Radhaa broke the spell I was under and helped to restore my sovereignty and spiritual gifts. Radhaa expertly walked me through the stickiness of the dark programming that had been holding me hostage for most of my life. With Brigid as our Goddess Guide, we went into a few parallel timelines. We focused on a timeline where I lived in the Renaissance. Here I was fully expressed as an educated, classy, desirable woman who was a singer and author. I could see that these were some of the exact qualities I had been craving to share more in my current reality.

Out of jealousy and spite, my "current mother" had thrown me in a dungeon and cast some pretty evil sorcery upon my consciousness.

She was something akin to a Soul Stalker and had been mind-controlling me throughout many dimensions. Brigid released me from all the places where I had been tied up, around my ankles, hands, and neck.

Radhaa has an incredibly compassionate heart and a laser-sharp awareness of the underpinnings of what is really going on. No other healer had been able to get to the depth of this issue for me before. For a few days – a week after our session, I just allowed much of the negativity and toxicity to unravel throughout my nervous system.

I rarely had if ever felt my SOVEREIGNTY before and wanted to relish in it. Brigid had performed energetic surgery on my throat chakra, so I took one entire day to be in silence as I integrated and called back all the lost pieces of my Divine Light.

Amazingly, we were also able to contact my Twin Flame, who was hunky, funny, and loving. Knowing he was there as part of my spirit team helper to restore my heart and soul to its fullest integrity to fulfill my mission successfully.

Right away, I began to feel my own bubbly soulful signature, which is, was, and always has been, an Angelic bright light. In the days following, I noticed that I was beginning to emit my own purified energetic frequency out into my world.

What a miracle! It was as if a black magic spell had been lifted. There are no words to express the gratitude I have for the gifts that Radhaa provides. She's a truly remarkable healer. If you've ever felt trapped or persecuted, then this is the kind of energy healing that will help you get to the root of blockages. Tap into your Goddess whom you feel connected to and allow Radhaa to be your guide to recover lost aspects of your true self.

Holy White Fire

Goddess Activations™ is a gift from the Divine Realm facilitated via Radha. It can be seen as an initiation for the woman who is ready to release deep-seated karmic patterning.

I'm excited to expand into my healing abilities and capacities as a modern-day Success and Destiny Priestess and Shaman. Once I recognized that I held a chalice full of Holy White Fire, I wanted to understand this divine empowerment.

I discovered that White Light is the original spark of purity, the beginning, the essential goodness. This flame has burned in the hearts of many wisdom keepers for eons and burned in the torches of Goddess temples and the hearths of priestesses. It's an eternal flame that cannot be put out by anyone or anything. In truth, the White Light is stronger than any illusion of darkness.

This White Flame Energy is part of the reprogramming to remember our connection to Mother Earth, to the Goddesses, and to heal the 2500 years old wound of being wiped out of religious history. Perhaps most importantly, we can activate our purpose, tap into our Shakti and transform the past, present, and future when we align with this sacred white flame.

Now that I am a Pillar of Light for The Goddess of Brigid - I choose to walk in beauty, love, and majesty from this day forward.

As a result of my Goddess Activations™, I was inspired to express more of my authentic voice through my writing. I want to share my poems that emerged as part of my transformational journey with Radhaa and Goddess Brigid.

MICHELLE L. CASTO

~ CONTRIBUTING WRITER ~

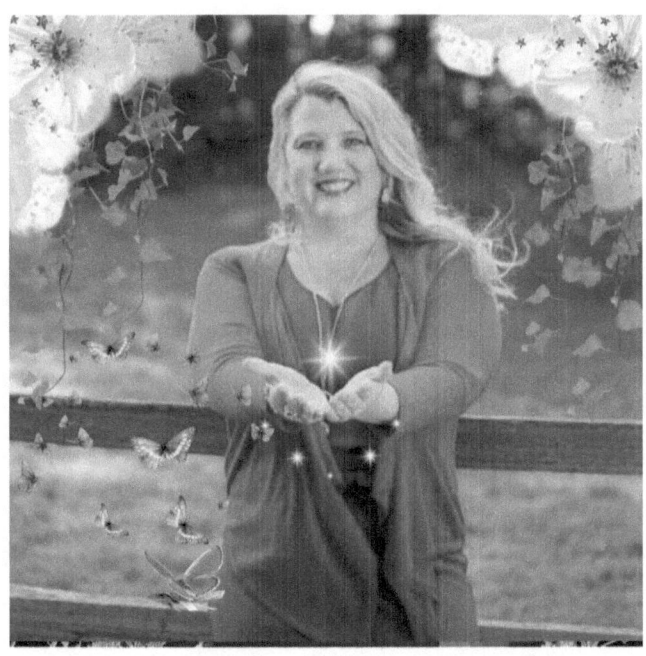

Michelle L. Casto is the Founder of Finding Your Wealthy Queendom - for change agents and leaders to bring forward the New Paradigm of Success. Speaker, Spiritual Energy Healer, and Purpose & Success Coach. Her mission is to empower awakening people to discover and live their greatest Destiny.

Overcoming her childhood neglect and emotional trauma, she developed Quantum Success Energetics, a transformative energy healing method works at the light body level to release hidden barriers and unwind underlying stressful thought patterns.

Expert in transformation, she provides a sacred healing space to activate the clarity, self-love, and confidence to achieve "Soulful Success." Prolific author of The Destiny Discovery: Find Your Soul's Path to Success and Heart Empowerment for Empaths.

Discover the difference between letting life happen to you and creating your life on purpose. It changes everything!

www.CoachMichelleCasto.com

CHAPTER 18

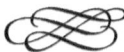

MARY MAGDALENE GODDESS ACTIVATIONS™

Blossom Rountree

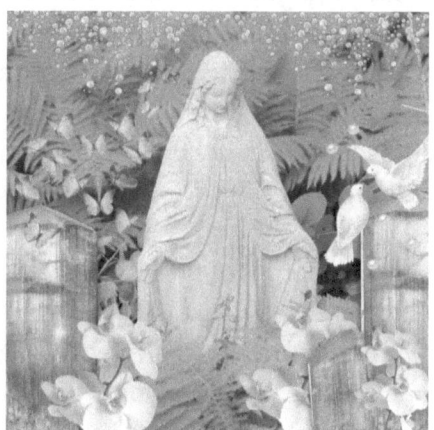

I chose Mary Magdalene for my Goddess Activations because I had an experience reading a book written by a soul group member. I will not name the book here; however, it was transformative for me. It is a channeled book about Mary Magdalene (Miriam) and Jesus (Yeshua) and their soul group. This book had such a profound effect on me that I now believe that I lived during these times and was a student of the Goddess or even that I may be a part of their soul group. I say this with great humility and do not consider myself above or better than anyone else. Before reading this book, I had somewhat of a level of rejection for the concept of Jesus or Christ. The reason being that in my heart, I understood or had the inner knowing that God did not expect every human on earth to believe one specific way or they were doomed to hell and that we only have one life to come to this conclusion. I believe there are truths in all religions, but no religion has all of the answers. However, I can honestly say that I have fallen in love with Jesus and see the great beauty and sacrifice he made to bring the teachings to our planet during a very dense time in history. I believe him to be an Ascended Master and that a great portion of the Bible was purposefully left out to instill fear and control upon humanity.

Mary Magdalene is very misunderstood by most. In the Bible, she is portrayed as a whore or prostitute. But many believe and know, including me, that she is the feminine aspect of the Divine Counterpart of Yeshua or Jesus Christ. She is his equal, and this is the energy we are returning to, one of equality and unity of the masculine and feminine within and without. I believe that we are all awakening to our inner god/goddess energy. I am humbled and honored to assist in this process of anchoring these codes during this Great Awakening and time of Ascension.

Mary Magdalene was purposefully misconstrued in the Bible to disempower the feminine further. Just like the story of Adam and Eve. To become Christed means to carry the threefold flame of enlightenment. The Threefold Flame is blue, gold, and pink, representing Divine Wisdom, Divine Power, and Divine Love. We are all capable of achieving this to becoming Christed, and it is also known as our Buddha Nature. In the Bible, Jesus said, "Timeless truth, I tell you: whoever believes in me, those works which I have done he will also do, and he will do greater works than these, because I AM going to the presence of my father."

When I met my twin flame, I began experiencing joy for the first time in my life. True joy is such a pure blissful state of being. But at the same breath, I became angry with every other man in my life because I realized what greatness men were capable of, and I believed they had not chosen or were probably more likely unable to express this in themselves for one reason or another. I wondered how if men are truly capable of this gentleness, love, and compassion, why were they not choosing to be that?

At the same time, I looked at my own life to figure out where my anger was coming from. My grandmother hated men because of her life experiences of being heartbroken, always being second to her brother, and coerced to marry someone she did not love. Of course, this dislike and distrust of men were passed on to me through my mother as well. I was raised by lesbian mothers and had an abusive relationship with my father. I do understand how this hatred towards the masculine is perpetually carried down through our ancestry lines. But these are all stories that we have lived through for one reason or another. What if we could let go of these stories and begin to see the men in our lives in a different light? How would that shift our lives, our realities?

My answer to this question now is because of fear. Fear to be who we truly are. We all have so many traumas and wounds to heal on a collective level, and I have great compassion for what the men have had to carry all these generations. What if we could learn to love and accept our inner masculine and feminine aspects completely?

Why Goddess Activations™?

I recently became more abundantly aware that I have difficulty hiding and remaining in the shadows because of fear of being seen for who I really am. I have fears about not wanting to be seen or heard.

It is one of the main reasons I chose to do the Goddess Activations. I knew that it would push me out of my comfort zone quickly, that I would be forced to be seen, and that it would help me achieve my next alignment and leveling up. I am so grateful to Radhaa Nilia for this beautiful and perfectly timed experience.

My Session With Radhaa

During the activation, Radhaa could clear and collapse the timelines where I had lived lives of persecution for my gifts. She released the martyr energy that I had carried throughout all of my lifetimes back to its origin. She was also able to release all the energy around feeling like I was not enough. I had not discussed this with her at all, and it was the energy that I had been working on to clear.

Radhaa is extremely intuitive and clairvoyant, just to name a few of her many gifts. As we began the session, she ground my energy and moved up through my crown into the heart of the Creator. She asked me to release one layer of anything that I am ready to let go of, including any fears. I immediately felt very expansive and heart-opening. She asked if I worked with any specific guides and if calling them in for assistance was ok. I said yes, of course. Then she brought in the Blue Avians from Lyra to join me because I believe this to be my origin. She let me know that only higher energies of love can come into this space, into the heart of the Creator. She said whoever comes in is an aspect of my higher Self or past lives.

Many Egyptian beings, including Isis, began showing up to assist with the clearings and activations. She said that many multi-dimensional aspects of myself were coming forward, including my higher Self. I immediately saw magenta and could feel the love radiating when Mary Magdalene entered the space with us. Mary Magdalene is trained in the ways of the Goddess by Isis, so I was delighted and humbled that she was also there to assist me during this activation.

Radhaa asked what energies I wanted to clear and release during the session that I believed would help me anchor these codes. I told her that I had experienced a lot of shame in my life and in my twin connection that I had been working on and clearing myself. I told her that I also believed clearing this would be important to hold the Mary Magdalene pillar and codes. I had a lot of fear of being seen or visible. Radhaa asked me where I believed the shame and these fears of being seen came from, and I told her that I felt like it was past lives of persecution and needing to hide who I am. It is very deep inside me. She tuned into my lifetimes of shame and fear of visibility.

Mary Magdalene assisted Radhaa on collapsing timelines needed for me to come forward.

Timeline #1: Radhaa said several Egyptian timelines needed collapsing. She said it was a traumatic and brutal time, and what happened in Egypt was the same as what happened in Greece in that the feminine was running the temples. They were in charge of the sacred rituals. And then, at some point, the men got very jealous of the feminine divine power. And so they tossed them out, and they did a takeover. It was very traumatic, brutal. And it was not inclusive. The women were eradicated out of the temple. She added that I was a very devoted priestess, the trauma that I felt disconnected me, and being ripped away from that devotional energy had stopped the flow of my divine feminine energy.

She asked if I had any memories or anything and came forward with it. I told her of a dream I had when my twin and I were physically together. "I dreamed that we were both inside the temples or pyramids, and I was teaching or guiding people on teleportation." I have always felt this lifetime that if I could have one superpower, I wanted to teleport. I do believe that we are heading towards this someday soon. We were so advanced then and had fallen into 3D. Radhaa added, "We're on the upswing back to higher consciousness, thank God. But that's why this work with these activations in bringing the pillars of light back is vital because it's helping to anchor in that feminine. The reason why the world is so imbalanced, as you know, is because we're not in alignment with the feminine."

Similarly, Magdalene was completely shamed and shunned. The values have been misconstrued, and they've been distorted. And so this is why we have to re-code everything the distortion that has been done. It was like a virus, and it has distorted every facet and everything, including technology. Yes, we're going back to that divine timeline, and we're going back to the truth, says Radhaa.

Then Radhaa reactivated some of the sacred remembering. She asked the Goddess to bring back online some of my sacred memories of being in the temples and activated my gifts, including the knowledge and dreams that I would be able to access them in Divine time. She activated them back into my DNA, RNA, consciousness, and unconscious mind.

Timeline #2: The next timeline presented for clearing was in New England. She referred to it as the witchy times. She said I was super pissed off and feisty. We had a good chuckle about that. She said this timeline of the witch hunts helped create the trauma that made it difficult to own my gifts in other lives. Radhaa also released all of the negative attention energy that I received during these times.

Mary Magdalene continued to assist Radhaa in choosing which timelines needed to be cleared.

Timeline #3: Another timeline that came into focus was when I was a farmer's wife. I apparently felt extremely suppressed, hidden, and powerless. A silent torment of living in a man's world and pumping out the babies, not having the opportunity to have my own voice and shine in my own light and truth. I was apparently very resentful and angry in this life. She said that I felt abandoned by the Divine. I can see how this also played out in my current life. While she was clearing it, I could physically feel it draining out of me through the bottom of my feet. It was a very strong sensation. Once cleared, an orange butterfly showed up and notified her that it was time for me to take my wings back. I saw it as a sign of transforming from the caterpillar or chrysalis stage to finally becoming the butterfly and taking flight. Next, the martyr template energy was released and collapsed throughout all timelines in all time-space and dimensions back to the point of origin. I am so grateful for this as well. After that was completed, she had me take a deep breath and release the energy out of my cells. Then she asked me to take three deep breaths bringing new energy back into my being. She had me say out loud, "it's safe for me to shine, my gifts are valuable, and it's safe for me to be seen in this world."

Now it was time to connect with Mary Magdalene. Radhaa said she wanted to connect face to face, heart, to heart, soul to soul with me. She placed a red rose into my heart to help me learn to receive. Then she placed a rose in each of my chakras, instructed me to connect with the rose energy daily, and told me I would find new inspiration and healing energy. With each deep breath, we released the old paradigm energy. The Rose lineage is now reactivated within me into my whole being for full embodiment. She sent 100,000 roses to me, and as they began blooming, infinite blooming over and over, this created the release of any old toxicity and old paradigm energy.

Mary Magdalene, through Radhaa, activated me back to my original soul blueprint and re-coded me, blooming back my gifts and truths. She reminded me that I am love and the beloved, and that divine union is happening within me. And that's why I am going through this challenging separation. I must activate and recalibrate my own inner union. She said that it is reactivating Christ's consciousness on earth, and that Mary Magdalene was really honored that I chose her because she also chose me. I felt moved to tears by the sheer gravity and importance of restoring these sacred codes to our beautiful planet earth and to me. Mary Magdalene told Radhaa that she would work with her afterward to tell her specific rituals that I need to do to keep my vibration high enough to hold this light in my pillar. She said the truth does not need to be shouted from the rooftops. It can just be anchored into us as a living vessel of the living Goddess energy, and that carrying this is very important at this time and will require that I perform certain rituals to maintain this new vibration.

Mary Magdalene said that I was very loved, proud of me and that she wanted me to stand tall and stand in my light to remember that this is not my first initiation and this current time we are in is probably one of the most important timelines of all time, which I could not agree with more.

"We are anchoring in the original codes and divine blueprint. That we are at a critical mass point."

The Goddess stands within me and behind me, and there is a legion of divine angels standing with me. I must do my work and continue to share it even when I feel as though people are tired of hearing about it because it helps people Ascend. She instructed me to surround myself with the rose energy daily and plant a small rose bush with my affirmations as an offering to the earth, the rose lineage, and my higher Self.

My energy felt so expansive and light. Mary Magdalene told her that part of my mission would be working with men, the masculine energy, to help heal their hearts and assist them during the ascension. She added; I would be holding retreats and doing drumming circles around the campfire. I am so honored to be able to serve the masculine in this way. To help them heal their beautiful sacred hearts.

This past year I have acquired three drums that I knew would become part of my mission work but had not yet been shown how that would manifest until now. I am looking forward to seeing how this energy will continue to grow inside me as I continue to embody the Rose Lineage.

Yesterday, I awoke to feel this balance between the masculine and feminine polarities. I believe I experienced some activations and energy healings during my sleep. I could almost feel the two energies on either side of me, but also outside of my body, like poles or maybe even columns of light. During the activation with Radhaa, I also experienced seeing the color magenta, which I believe to be the third energy created from the inner and outer union. I know that my inner union is happening more rapidly thanks to this beautiful, life-changing activation. I am coming back into wholeness within and without.

Words of Encouragement

If we can look at all the parts of ourselves that we feel less than and love them anyway, we can become whole again. What if we could accept the fact that we are capable of everything we could ever imagine? That the possibilities are endless!? That the only thing that limits us is our minds and belief systems? What if we started questioning where we even came up with those beliefs in the first place? What if we truly believed that nothing was standing in the way of being healed of whatever disease, syndrome, or ailment that may cause us suffering? Could we let go of all attachment to our suffering? All attachment to the negative and positive things that we may believe we gain from being "sick"? Could you accept your healing in this "now moment?" Could you accept that you are an infinite being with limitless possibilities and fully capable of healing yourself in this present moment, in this now? When you are in this "now moment," you can accept what is and let go of any suffering that you believe yourself to be experiencing. In this moment is where creation is made possible.

The more you practice and become aware of each moment and just be present with yourself, the more your life will transform. It will allow you to let go of all attachments. You will become aware and conscious of the fact that you do not need anything outside of yourself. You are whole and complete, just as you are. You will no longer desire anything outside of yourself. By doing this paradoxically, life will become a beautiful flowing river of opportunity and grace. You will step into and align with your soul's guidance. You will surrender your will to the will of Divine Source/ God. You will experience states of pure bliss regularly, and you will radiate that out into the world. It is how we raise the collective consciousness of humanity. It is how we anchor heaven on earth. It is our one true ultimate mission.

Go within. Everything we need exists inside of us. All of the answers that we are seeking can be found within ourselves. When we can quiet the mind and listen to our inner knowing, we will find all the answers we have been searching for. We will no longer need anything outside of ourselves. We will no longer need anything or anyone to complete us or make us whole. All of the great masters and teachings have been trying to tell us this in one form or another. When we go within and heal ourselves and do our inner work, it also heals our world. By healing ourselves, we heal our reality. To do this inner work, we must first realize that we are not our thoughts. We are the witness to these thoughts. Once we can disconnect from our thoughts and realize it is our ego talking and running the show, we can then ask the ego to step aside and begin consciously creating our reality instead of creating it from our subconscious wounds and traumas experienced throughout our lives.

God/Source is pure unconditional love. Fear is the opposite of love, the opposite of God. Fear is the darkness that we find ourselves currently experiencing and living in. In this 3D duality world, fear is the only thing keeping us in separation from God. Are you willing to let go of your fear? Are you willing to begin to consciously examine what you are really afraid of and then take action towards letting it all fall away so that you can return to the pure loving being that you are? "Nothing to fear, except fear itself." It truly is. I believe no truer words were ever spoken.

It is what Mary Magdalene has come forward to ask of you. She asks you to wake up and remember who you are and embrace your God/Goddess-self, your inner Divine Spark, to reach inner union within and help anchor Heaven on Earth for all of humanity.

Radhaa created such a beautiful space and sacred container for these Goddess Activations™ to be brought through. I could feel so strongly the immense love and gratitude during the process.

BLOSSOM ROUNTREE

~ CONTRIBUTING WRITER ~

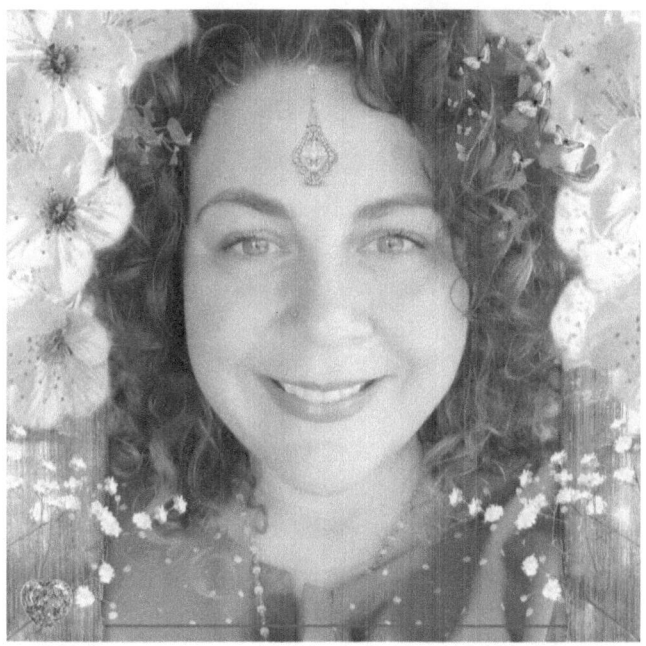

Blossom is a lightworker, a twin flame here to help raise the collective consciousness during this Great Awakening. She offers spiritual guidance during this ascension process and practices Emotion Code, Body Code, and Biomagnetic Pair Therapy. She also offers a technique to heal the subconscious mind that has split off due to trauma and bring it back into wholeness. She serves by assisting people in raising their frequency which allows a shift in their awareness and leads to the ability to transcend physical ailments. blossomingoneness@gmail.com

Saying:

"What happened to the Divine Feminine? Why has She apparently disappeared from Judaism, Christianity, and Islam? In the Gnostic Gospels, we learn that Mary Magdalene was probably the closest disciple of the Christos, the one whom the Master taught the most arcane esoteric wisdom. She was and is the representation of all wisdom. The male apostles of the Christos demonstrated both their jealousy and respect for the wisdom and position of
Mary Magdalene."

~ Laurence Galian

CHAPTER 19

JOURNEY TO THE GODDESS

Radhaa Nilia

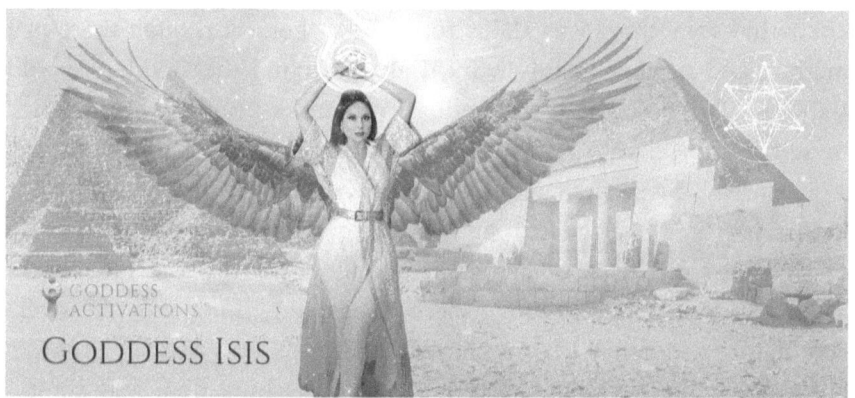

GODDESS HEALING HOUSE

After many years of training in no less than a dozen holistic modalities, I finally opened my healing house in Hollywood Hills. As fate had it, I moved to this magical little home on Decente Drive off Laurel Canyon. It had huge windows, tons of trees and enveloped me with healing vibrations, and I felt embraced in its warmth. The backyard was a view of the city, but it felt like a forest. This is where I first set up a sacred healing space. It had one room that was whispering to me, 'I am meant to be a healing room.' I could have used it for anything, a spare office, a wardrobe, but I knew that it had it's purpose and I was in alignment with that purpose.

My mother and I spent a week hand-painting the room in the most soothing salmon pink. We had a salmon-colored wearable art gallery for many years, and the color just seemed to bring healing energy to all who entered our door. So we rolled healing vibrations into the walls to hold space for those who walked through our sacred space.

The room's only purpose was for healing sessions. My mother and I both had clients coming daily, it just felt like the Goddess House of Healing. The energy reverberated throughout the Hills. That's the beauty about energy work, mantras, prayers, healing. When you do it repeatedly in a certain place, it creates a patterning in the frequencies and a healing portal. And that's how I felt living there. I adored and cherished my clients, feeling butterflies of joy when they came over, I knew that something was about to shift for them. Although there is a method and rhythm in this work, I always found the Goddess would lead me. That kept the work feeling fresh and a beautiful surprise for myself and my clients. I was grateful that through word of mouth, my work spread. Since my clients and neighborhood were entertainment industry folk, I started to get invited to Hollywood Studios to do sessions for actresses or actors, and once I was on the lot, others asked to work with me too. Everyone has something they are overcoming or need help with, myself included.

Progress. Each Goddess would bring something new, and I felt I was getting fast-tracked in my Goddess essence, energy, and studies in real-time with each Goddess as I worked with my clients. My experiences have provided me the strength to move forward with the quest for a deeper meaning in life while being in service. In doing so, my process kept me going into assisting others through the method of Goddess Activations™.

Over the years, I continued to work with both women and men, and I embodied my work as a Goddess Guide. More women from all walks of life gravitated towards me, eager to make their journey to the Goddess towards their healing and transformations. I have seen my clients experience the shift they needed from the Goddess Activations™. These changes include self-empowerment, more self-confidence, personal fulfillment, and enigmatic presence, a sense of pride in sharing who she is, and the ability to manifest what she wants in life — love, healing and abundance.

"The fear of speaking her truth has caused a silent pain and suffering for so many women."

The freedom to speak one's truth and express oneself is vital in living one's life. Realizing this unbearable need for truth, women seek answers. Many women these days are willing to do the deep healing work required towards their liberation.

Activate Your Inner Priestess

The Goddesses are arising at the forefront of human consciousness. They are here to initiate and challenge the feminine into our benevolent feminine power. It is time to reclaim your feminine leadership that starts with your heart.

I created the Pillars of Light, a temple for you to walk into and embody your inner Goddess and be your inner Priestess. In this most difficult threshold we are crossing in this world, from dark to light, we are being asked to be courageous and stand as living Pillars of Light.

The Goddesses are urging us to cultivate all we are at this time. In our temple, we invite you to deepen your spiritual core practices and mystical skills that we offer at the Pillars of Light temple at Goddess Code Academy. When you awaken your sense of discipline, commitment, and accountability in practices that strengthen the body, mind, and spirit, it assists you to build your inner foundation, stabilize your core, and strengthen your capacity to be of service to yourself and the changing world.

As conscious beings, I know you're longing to be a holder of love and light yearning to be a benevolent Priestess leader. We are the sacred witness, the bearer of creating life in our wombs. The divine feminine is being called to come together, stand for what's righteous, to awaken our divine gifts as the conduit of love and light as Priestesses of Goddess temples. Once awakened in consciousness, we can never again tolerate the mental illness behind this planetary destruction.

The Goddesses are here to provide the groundwork for staying more present, more grounded, more courageous, and more available in these very challenging times. Our world is splitting apart. The patriarchal ideals, systematic oppression are beginning to show their dark shadows in many areas of our reality, from governments withholding basic human rights and implementing undeniable control. It is all coming up to the surface for humanity to see in plain sight. The time we are in does not allow anything to hide in the shadows any longer. Everything is being pushed to the surface to be seen, leading people across the globe to stand for their human rights.

In understanding the depth of how patriarchal control has touched every fabric of our lives and society at large, we too can see how the Goddess can also counter this with her healing love, presence, and blessings.

The Goddess is here to serve us in dismantling the old paradigm. She is here to usher us into divine remembrance during this deeply chaotic but important timeline in the history of our planetary transformation. The Goddesses call us to stand for our highest truth, beliefs, and belief in ourselves, our wombs, and our feminine wisdom.

As we become more aware of what is truly taking place on our beautiful planet, there are agents of destructive forces against humans, plants, and animals, and we are being urgently awakened by our relationship with our star-Earth Mother for our species to exist.

In America, chemtrails are seen daily across the skies. Our air is constantly being sprayed with toxic chemicals. At the same time, our precious water is being disturbed by toxic chemicals from fracking, and all that poison from fracking gets to our underground tunnels, leaking and leading to our ocean filled with life. The garbage, plastics everywhere, and more pollution seem to have no end. The Goddesses are awakening us to become spiritual warriors and to say NO more.

It's easy to forget, but to remember is crucial because this is the greatest fight we ever encounter on the face of the Earth --- a fight for all lives; humanity, animals, and plants -- from the land, ocean, and air, we are faced with challenges to stand for all of us, and the survival of our future generations to live freely, joyfully and abundantly. We can no longer turn away our sights nor cover our ears to helplessly not recognize that this mindless destruction is tearing us apart. The stake is very high. The control over humanity in outpouring of media lies to keep humans dumb and dumber. But it has gone too far.

And here we stand sister, at the edge of Kali Yuga, the end of darkness just before we step into Satya Yuga, the age of light, truth, and peace--here we are given a cosmic opportunity to straighten out the inversions that have been placed within us in all aspects of ourselves and this world. This may all sound like too much, scary, hard, and impossible. But the Goddesses are here to remind you that you are the one you've been waiting for. It's time to awaken from this nightmare! The Priestess temple is here to help you ground yourself through rituals and anchor the Goddess light on Earth.

A new grid of divine feminine light is needed now more than ever in every part of this planet. A woman initiated in the Goddess path by activating her Goddess Code, becomes a Holy vessel, and contributes as a Priestess of the new paradigm.

When you choose to become a Priestesses, you will be one of the changing winds that can blow away the impending chaos and curses projected to our star Mother and her beings. We can collectively turn the evil ways around as we participate in our gathering prayers rituals and connect more and more of our sisters. We are stronger together. Let's come together with the tsunami of devotion to the Goddesses to support humanity. Sisters, we are in between timelines–a crucial and a very important one because there is no other time than the time NOW! Cosmic help will come sooner than later!

Saying:

"There is nothing stronger than a broken woman who has rebuilt herself.

~Hannah Gadsby

GET TRAINED IN GODDESS ACTIVATIONS™

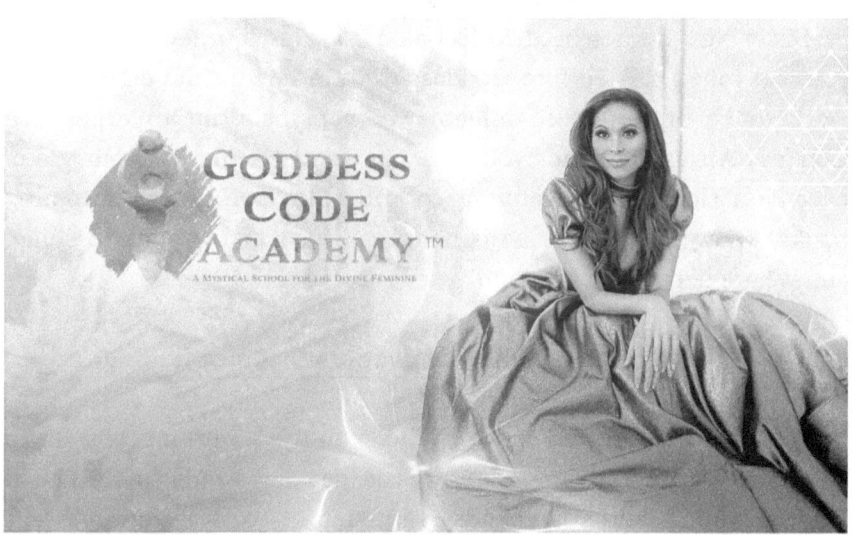

*I*f you are seeking guidance, mentorship, or training, I am here for you. I so enjoy working with women in the training aspect of this work. Some women want to learn for themselves, and others wish to be a practitioner of this modality.

Shine as A Pillars of Light

It is time to reignite the Pillars of Light within those who are ready to receive. An invitation from the divine to deeply fall in love with yourself all over again. Get to know the Goddesses. There is joy in discovering the Goddess's gifts, guidance, and the freedom from bondage and limitations of our indoctrinated beliefs. Goddess energy can spark back up stagnant energies that need recharging. It is never too late for a woman to be the woman of her dreams!

As you know, I also curate holistic books in which you are invited to be a part of our collaborative book series. Storytelling is one of the most powerful ways to be relatable, share information and experience the joy of co-creating for a higher purpose. That is why it is so important that we heal and create.

Sister, you do not need to feel alone on this journey called life. If you feel called to step into Goddess Code Academy and embody this work to be of service to others, whether you want to experience Goddess Activations™ for yourself, and stand up and use your voice, become a Goddess Activator or contribute to one of our upcoming books, know that your tribe is here for you. It's your time to shine, and we are here to support you!

A part of this Goddess Activations™ is storytelling

I'm a keeper of sacred stories. When you work with me, you get to share your story with me. Later, if you decide to publish them, I'm here for you. I hold your hands every step of the way towards self-empowerment. I am your Goddess coach and Goddess healer. Like these women in the Pillars of Light book, they could fully self-express themselves through storytelling after they experienced Goddess Activations™.

Either way, you'll receive a ton of personal healing just by working in the temple of the Goddesses with me. After you've read these pages, you can always reach out to me if you find this interesting.

I offer certification courses

You can start with one Goddess Archetype or learn them all. I start by introducing the concept of the Goddess Archetypes and the process of Goddess Activations™. You will then explore the Goddess and start tracking your own experiences that will guide you in the process of activating the Goddess Code™. By immersing transmissions, you will have the tools you need for life to activate your highest purpose and your intuitive powers to call anything you desire into your life.

The Goddesses were once revered and given space to rule the hearts and minds of ancient times benevolently. That is why it is essential to bring back the original integrity of the Pillars of Goddess

Light through Goddess Activations™. We are at the great evolutionary shift of the ages that is upon us, the Golden Age. Your wisdom, power, and magic are honored and greatly needed at this time on Earth.

Now is the time

"Liberate yourself from the chains of limitation and remember who you truly are."

The time has come for you to recollect and encode gifts you possess to transform your destiny and awaken your legacy we are here to create together. Courageously reclaim the crown of your sovereignty on the throne of your inner authority to benefit all beings everywhere. It is time for you to rise as a living embodied Goddess.

"The clarion call is here for you to receive the mantle of your divine inheritance and to lead with empowered feminine grace."

∼

Saying:

"Feel like a Goddess, think like a Goddess, manifest like a Goddess, activate your inner Goddess."

~Radhaa Nilia

RADHAA NILIA
CREATRIX OF GODDESS ACTIVATIONS™

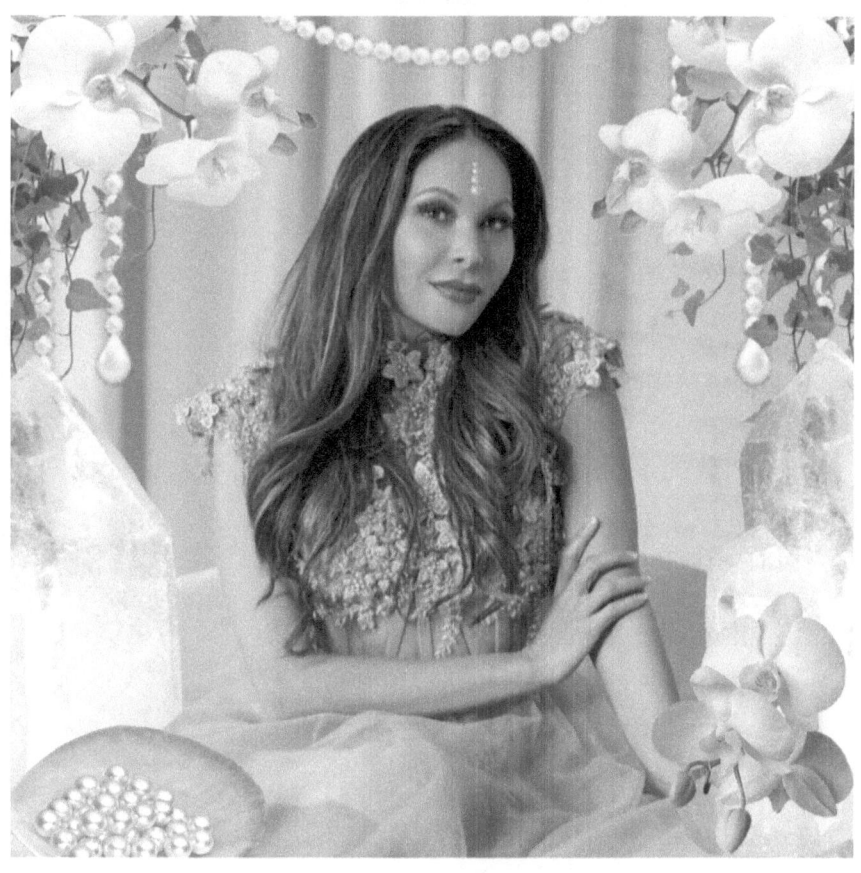

Radhaa Nilia is a Feminine Leader, Creatrix of Goddess Code Academy: A mystical school for the Divine Feminine. An online temple where she teaches her original modality, Goddess Activations™.

"Radhaa supports visionary feminine leaders into bridging the intangible teachings of the Goddess into the physical realms of Life, Business, and Prosperity."

As the Guardian of Goddess Activations™ and a Priestess of Pillars of Light temple, Radhaa is one of today's most up-and-coming speakers and teachers on the Goddess Archetypes. Please join our mailing list to receive upcoming invitations on events at: www.GoddessCodeAcademy.com

Radhaa Nilia's Credentials, Training and Certifications

Founder of Goddess Code Academy
Creatress of Goddess Activations™
Certified DNA ThetaHealing Instructor for Beginners
Certified Advanced DNA ThetaHealing Instructor
Certified Manifestation & Abundance Coach
DNA ThetaHealer Beginners Practitioner
Advanced DNA ThetaHealer Practitioner
Certified Level 1 Akashic Reader, Healer & Practitioner
Certified Level 2 Akashic Reader, Healer & Practitioner
Certified Lemurian Code Healer
Certified Infinite Cosmic Records Healer
Certified Raindrop Therapist
Certified Relationship Coach
Certified Level 1 Aka Dua Transmission
Certified Level 2 Aka Dua Transmission
Certified Red Tent Facilitator
Certified Access Bars Practitioner
Certified Ordained Minister
Graduate of Art of Meditation
Certified Ho'oponopono Practitioner
Certified Golden DNA Practitioner
Certified Practitioner of Jseals, Unnatural Seals & Implant Removal

Certified Christ Activation Practitioner
Completed Producers Program at UCLA
Advanced Communication Course: Power to Create
Advanced Communication Course: Access To Power
Team Leadership Program
Founder of Radhaa Publishing House
Recipient of Best Director Award for Feature Film Hope Cafe
Recipient of Best Actress Award for short Film Freight Train
Recipient of State of California Senate Recognition for Leadership and Contribution of Service in the Community.

As a Goddess Activator and Business Woman, Radhaa's otherworldly gifts have guided her into successfully creating Radhaa Publishing House. A heart-centered Publishing company focusing on collaborative books and offers creative writing programs, and one-to-one coaching for up-and-coming authors. The Awakening Starseeds book series is the first original Starseeds collaborative book of its kind and is an ongoing series. Soon after many more heartfelt and real life stories are being recorded at Radhaa Publishing House as books for you to be a part of. Please join our mailing list to receive upcoming information about our books and programs.

Find out more at:

www.RadhaaPublishingHouse.com
www.GoddessCodeAcademy.com
www.RadhaaNilia.net

Saying:

"We make your writing dreams come true!"

~Radhaa Publishing House

ABOUT RADHAA PUBLISHING HOUSE

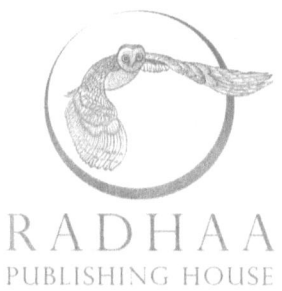

BECOME AN AUTHOR
BECOME A CONTRIBUTING WRITER

Radhaa Publishing House is a holistic publishing company that focuses on helping heart-centered, mind-expanding, truth-telling authors get their work out into the world. Our focus is on collaborative book series and memoirs. We thrive on supporting our authors and contributing writers throughout this journey, empowering them to step into their divine and an authentic voice while sharing their truth with the world. We especially celebrate cultural diversity worldwide, and we believe in weaving international voices to come together.

How are we different?

Many collaborative publishing companies bundle the authors together so that they don't receive individual credit and acknowledgment. We make sure each Author is seen and heard and can be found easily. This has led to authors telling us that they have received more traffic and business and clients on their websites. In a sense, each of the Book we create is also like a Directory highlighting contributing writers unique offerings. This has been a win-win for the contributing writers and authors.

Here is what our authors have said about working with us:

"I felt totally supported. The best bit was feeling like being part of a loving family who wants you to be your best, do your best, and is there for you every step of the way. It also boosted my confidence as a writer. The collaborative nature of the project also made it way more fun than doing things alone".
   *- **Arrameia, Prague***

"Visibility was a big piece of me coming out of the spiritual closet, and I felt that Radhaa Publishing House has a high energy and integrity level. Both of which are important for light workers and Starseeds. The curators and authors are light workers. Radhaa Publishing House created this wonderful opportunity for many others to be a part of. I felt that they put their whole heart into making this happen even before, during, and after the book is published. It was a project that was totally supportive that made me feel safe to share myself and my story." **- Lalitah, Turkey**

"It was wonderful to work with Radhaa Publishing House. I saw the effort and perseverance the whole team has and the support system they have for all the authors. I have matured as an author from this experience. I was so inspired after writing my chapter in this book, Awakening Starseeds, that I wrote an entire book called The Great Awakening because I was deeply moved writing."
   - Leshara, Philippines

"My story was edited by Radhaa Publishing House, and let me tell you, it put me in tears! They made it better than the way I originally wrote and submitted it while keeping my story and voice true to its events. I read it, and tears just flowed because it was so good!" **- Cristal, Florida**

"I have published many books on Consciousness, empowerment subjects, and relationships, but I had never revealed raw, real stories of my life as with Awakening Starseeds. I wanted to join other authors writing personal stories, and Radhaa Publishing House made it simple and empowering to share from my heart in a real, raw way. This team of conscious, awesome Starseeds encourages a revolution to Awaken other Starseeds worldwide!" - **Stasia, Utah**

This is an opportunity to STEP OUT, SPEAK OUR TRUTHS. This is our time, an obligation to share and support others that live in fear and question their soul paths, their soul journey. - **Breda, Canada**

At **Radhaa Publishing House,** we are highly involved in the entire process and work personally with the authors to navigate authorship challenges.

Our authors are heart-centered, soul-driven, and ready to manifest their legacy. We acknowledge the courage and strength it takes to step out into the public eye, and our team is here to support you all the way.

Creating a book is a tedious process and requires persistence, patience, and perspective. There are many moving parts of the book that need attention, and our team knows how to work hard to ensure we can come through with flying colors for the final date of our release.

Step into your voice and be heard now! When you become a contributing writer or an author of Radhaa Publishing House, you empower yourself in a way you may have never experienced before. That's what our authors tell us. Claim your author power now!

"Be that change you wanted to be in our world!"

If you have a compelling story to share with the world, dream of being a published author, and wish to be a part of the Radhaa Publishing family, reach out to us.

"No other publishing company offers you in-house support the way that Radhaa Publishing House does. Your legacy awaits!"

To find out more information about how to Join us,
Become an Author or See our Upcoming Books, please visit our
Website at:
www.RadhaaPublishingHouse.com
Email: RadhaaPublishing@gmail.com

&

To Order a Signed Copies of our Books, visit our
Online Store: https://radhaanilia.net/shop/
Email us: RadhaaPublishing@gmail.com

BOOKS OF RADHAA PUBLISHING HOUSE

"You Make a Difference When You Support Our Holistic Books!"

2018-2019-2021 Books:
Awakening Starseeds: Shattering Illusions, Vol.1
Awakening Starseeds: Stories Beyond The Stargate, Vol. 2
Quan Yin Goddess Activations™ Healing Workbook

2022 Books:
Pillars of Light: Stories of Goddess Activations™ (Spring 2022)
Energy Healing & Soul Medicine (Late Spring, 2022)
Infinite Cosmic Records: Sacred Doorways to Healing & Remembering (Summer, 2022)
Awakening Starseeds: Dreaming into the Future, Vol. 3 (Fall, 2022)
Memoirs of a Galactic Goddess, 2nd Edition, Part 1 (Winter, 2022)

2023 Books:
Awakening Starseeds Vol. 4
Descendants of Lemuria: Memoir
Memoirs of a Galactic Goddess, 2nd Edition, Part 2

Where you can find Radhaa Publishing House Books:
Amazon.com — Barnes and Noble — Target
Walmart — Powell Books

*Get your Wholesale Copies at Radhaa Publishing House:
Minimum order is a dozen (12 books), shipping not included
Email: RadhaaPublishing@gmail.com

TO OUR READERS:

Dear Readers,

If you like our book, **"Pillars of Light: Stories of Goddess Activations™,"** please support us by leaving a review.

REVIEW us ONLINE at: Amazon.com. We cannot do this without your support!

Share this journey with us. With Love & Gratitude, thank you!

Pillars of Light Author,
    Radhaa Nilia

REVIEW THIS BOOK

PILLARS OF LIGHT: STORIES OF GODDESS ACTIVATIONS™

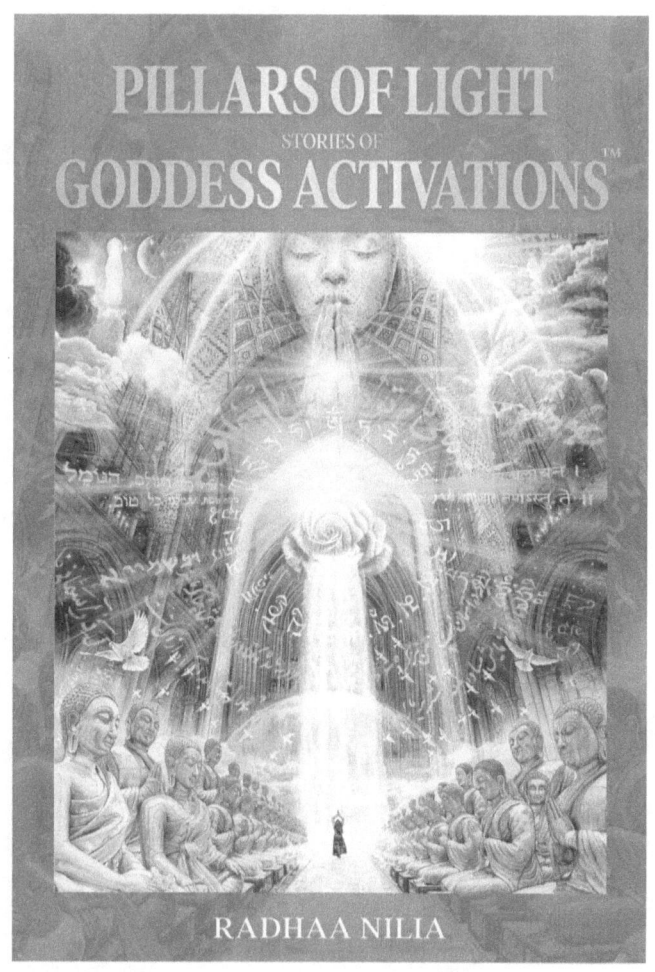

REVIEW us ONLINE at: Amazon.com.

www.ingramcontent.com/pod-product-compliance
Lightning Source LLC
Chambersburg PA
CBHW030148100526
44592CB00009B/172